DR. PUSHPA PANDEY 

Medicine
TO
MEDITATION

MY CANCER JOURNEY AND BEYOND

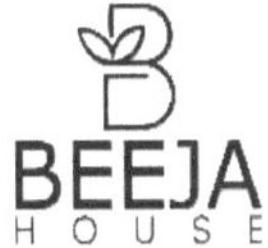

BEEJA
HOUSE

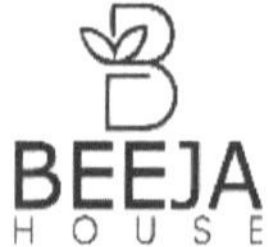

ISBN : 978-93-93635-82-2 (Paperback)

Published by: Beeja House

First Printing Edition 2022

Author Email: drpushpapandey@gmail.com

Foreword

It is an honour and pleasure to write this foreword to Medicine to Meditation - My cancer journey and beyond. When Dr. Pandey reached out and summarised the contents of this book, I was reminded of that significant day, way back in 1988 when I operated on Dadi Gulzar, a divine angel and the instrument of God for Breast Cancer. Her angelic and spiritual personality changed my life. I would find her always relaxed and smiling during her postoperative recovery. Instead of my asking her, it was she who would smilingly ask, "How are you, doctor ji?" It was the charisma of her spiritual power that transformed me into a "Double doctor", a term popular among Brahmakumaris indicating a doctor who not only treats physical illnesses but also of the spirit or soul, offering emotional support. After meeting this unique soul, who was the "Chariot of God", and getting introduced to Rajyoga, I realised being an eternal and a powerful soul and being introduced as a "Cancer Surgeon" was merely a role I was playing.

I have known Dr. Pushpa Pandey as a gynecologist and a spiritual doctor practising Rajyoga meditation for over 30 years.

Nevertheless, I had no clue about her challenging personal journey of "endometrial cancer". It is my observation that those who practice spirituality and meditation are able to handle traumatic personal experiences of going through treatment of life-threatening diseases like cancer better. They have a positive, strong mind which helps them recover faster.

"The mind alone is the friend of the self, and it alone is the foe of the self."

-Bhagavad Gita 6:5

Bhagavad Gita 6:5 reflects the basis of modern-day Mind-Body medicine. We often complain that others have given us sorrow, picturing them as our enemies, but the biggest enemy is our own minds. Our mind creates over 60,000 thoughts a day, most of them being wasteful and negative, leading to negative feelings, attitudes, and visions. We tend to suppress these feelings. This suppression may sow the seeds of some cancers and non-communicable diseases. Expression in the right way to the right person is necessary to be healthy. Most people may respond to a challenge of big 'C' as "Life is difficult", but with a positive attitude, these challenges can be converted into opportunities!

In this book, the role of meditation in healing life-threatening diseases like cancer is described very well. It was during the 1960s and 1970s when Dr. Herbert Benson demystified meditation, terming it as a "relaxation response", and helped it bring into the mainstream. Meditation is essentially the opposite of the "fight or flight" response to counteract the physiological effects of stress.

Meditation has been accepted as a good Mind-Body practice to reduce stress, anxiety, anger, and other negative emotions. An increasing number of physicians prescribe meditation for a large and growing number of conditions. Mind-body approaches like meditation, breathing exercises, and yoga take advantage of interactions between the mind and body to promote healing and health.

This interesting experience, shared by Dr. Pandey, is a practical spiritual guide that describes steps to prevent and heal cancer, and overcomes fear. The various tools and techniques described are a perfect blend of science and spirituality. She also describes how the invisible healing energy in the form of gratitude, forgiveness, and blessings helps in our lives every day. Doctors practising modern medicine in our country will be able to help and guide their patients to take care of these energies. They will radiate positive energy to the workplace, and to their patients and bring positive energy home for more happiness in their lives.

This book will not only comfort and inspire cancer survivors and their loved ones, but will be of unique support, especially for women in our society. The third section, which is the preventive part, is very useful for every woman who should undergo screening for cancers, which is lucidly described in question-answer format. I congratulate Dr. Pandey for this simple, practical, and informative guide to spreading health and happiness.

Dr. Ashok Mehta

Medical director and consultant surgeon, Brahma Kumaris Global Hospital managing hospital, Andheri West, Mumbai (India)

Chief of the department of oncology, Dr. Balabhai Nanavati Hospital, Mumbai (1975-2002)

Chief of Surgery: Head and Neck, Tata Memorial Hospital (1970-1998)

President, Medical wing, Brahma Kumaris

Contents

Acknowledgement

Thank you is not just a word, it's rather reciprocating energy of love that allows the heart to receive more of it.

First and foremost we would like to express our gratitude to the Supreme Surgeon, God, for the blessings, support and energy that He bestowed upon us for writing this book.

We would like to thank the following people for their contributions without which this book could never have been created. They have all been of great help either directly or indirectly.

Dr. Shyamji Rawat, Prof. in the cancer department of Government Medical College Jabalpur - India, who unconditionally supported throughout the journey of the disease and while penning this book.

Dr. Ashok Mehta for taking the time to go over the manuscript and for offering his advice.

The Brahma Kumaris family, especially BK Brijmohan Bhaiji, Additional Secretary-General of Brahma Kumaris, BK Dr. Banarsi Bhaiji, Dr. Preeti Jain, Dr. Shashi Khare, Dr. Kavita Singh, Dr. Nisha Sahu, Dr. Shobha

Gupta, Dr. Ashish Gupta, Ashish Pathak and BK Bhavana, for supporting in many ways.

My family members who stood by me in this divine cause.

The gracious angels who read through the rough drafts and provided valuable feedback to improve the book- Dwipa Shah, Nishi, Dr. Anita Mishra, Dr. Richa Baharani, Dr. Kirti Parasher, Dr. Premchand Dwivedi, Dr. Vasumati Upadhye, Sunita and Dr. SK Pandey.

The patients and colleagues for their blessings and for making us more experienced.

The known or unknown writers of the short stories and quotes included in this book.

We acknowledge the editors, Apoorva and Geetika Saigal from Beeja House for their motivational support and for giving valuable direction on written communication skills.

Last but not least, to all those who have helped us over the course but whose names we have failed to mention.

Introduction

"If your size of courage is double than the trouble, then your trouble will become a water bubble."

On Hope

I am presenting this book as a gynaecologist, a cancer survivor and a spiritualist to encourage and empower my fellow beings and the women community to lead a healthy and happy life. In my long medical career, I have observed that the fear of death is the first to hit when any serious disease like cancer strikes. Those who hear about the disease feel sorry for the patient and unknowingly transfer negative vibrations and feelings. It is well known that healing mainly depends on vibrational energy. Positive vibrations from the patient, their relatives and medical professionals, with proper medical treatment, have miraculous effects on healing. One of my main aims in writing this book is to convey that one can change the consequence of any disease by having hope and not a victim attitude.

Role of spirituality and meditation

The well-known karma philosophy is the universal causal law by which good or bad actions determine the future modes of an individual's existence. I have been a Rajyoga meditation practitioner since 1986 and kindness has been my virtue. Some would question why would I have this severe disease despite leading a good life! The karma philosophy explains why no one can be spared from any disease due to past karmic accounts.

Since my lifestyle was meditative, I thought my response to this disease should be positive and worthy to be an example for others. Through the course of the disease, I had the feeling that whatever is happening is for the best and that God has made me an instrument for the well-being of society. I dove deeper into spiritual healing and implemented the learnings in my everyday life. After seeing the positive effects, I have decided to continue those practices for the rest of my present life journey. Throughout my healing journey, I was happy, positive and accepted this disease as an opportunity. Therefore, another aim of this book is to bring you to the realization that we are spiritual beings and should learn meditation for holistic healing of the self, which also plays a complementary role in curing the disease. In this book, I describe a simple method of meditation that can be practised easily.

Why read this book?

All the aspects of physical, emotional and spiritual, all 3-in-1, health and healing are covered in this book. Most of the contributors to the book are meditators themselves. They have contributed only for Godly service with no personal or professional gain. The last chapter on "Breast Awareness" is written by a famous onco-surgeon, Dr. Preeti Jain who is one of the few female senior surgical oncologists in India and a meditator. All the pen and ink illustrations are made by Jyoti Pandey, a software engineer in Microsoft USA and a Rajyoga meditation practitioner. In addition to the pictures, we have also added a few short stories to understand the subject matter more clearly.

Learning from my mistakes

Often we are too busy to grasp signals from God. Committing the mistake of not grasping those signals makes us make them even more. It is wise to learn from others' mistakes. The book focuses on the mistakes I committed and the lessons learned from a medical point of view. It is important to understand 'normal' and 'abnormal' menstruation during menopause, all of which are explained in this book.

Prevention is better than cure

To prevent common types of female cancers, there are certain screening methods that everyone should undergo regularly. All the essential screening methods that I learned in my personal and long medical experience of forty years have been covered. This book is divided into three sections. The first section talks about my story, mistakes and learning experience during my tryst with cancer. The second covers the spiritual tools that I used for my healing. The third section lists preventive and screening strategies to keep the uterus healthy and covers breast awareness. This section is presented in an interesting Q&A format. FAQs from our public sessions for women have also been covered.

Welcome to your feedback

Feedback is a gift. I would love to hear your feedback on this book. Please do write if you find the book helpful or have any questions. To learn about Rajyoga meditation, you can browse the Brahma Kumaris Youtube channel or visit a centre near you. I feel enlightened and immensely satisfied after finishing this book. Enjoy the book!

Dr. Pushpa Pandey
drpushpapandey@gmail.com

Section 1

My Story

"See your struggles. Keep yourself open to Him to receive His signals."

Selfless contribution to society is considered a very noble deed. Since childhood, I have tried to find meaning in everything I do and make it worthwhile to others, directly or indirectly. Cancer in my life was a blessing giving me an opportunity to contribute and explore a new dimension. This section talks about some sweet and sour experiences in my healing journey. The sole intention to consolidate these learnings is to spread awareness about the disease and share a new way to discover newer aspects of life.

Present-day lifestyle and modernisation have led to an increase in lifestyle diseases, one of which is emerging as "cancer". Being a gynaecologist, I have centred the focus of this book on cancers of the female reproductive system. The most common type of cancer of the female reproductive system in the USA is "uterine (endometrial) cancer", the one I had. Its rates are concerningly on the rise in India too. In the following chapters of this section, I share my healing journey of endometrial cancer from illness to wellness.

"Where there is life, there's hope"

- Marcus Tullius Cicero

Chapter 1

My Journey from Illness to Wellness

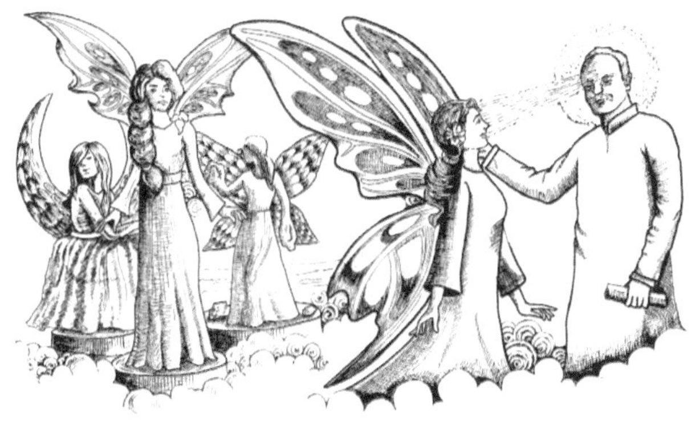

(Fig 1.1)

It was a peaceful night in March 2017 when I had a revelation. A dream was forewarning me about the impending challenges I was about to face.

As I lay in bed with my eyes closed, I saw a bright golden place, full of light and shimmer. Everything looked so pious and pure. The aureate light had enveloped the atmosphere making it look surreal. It was a beautiful angelic place and the moment I stepped forward, I was awestruck by the expanse of the place. I stood there, lost and numb. There were various statues of different people — men, women, old, and young and amid those statues, my eyes fell on one piece that was being carefully sculptured by a man dressed in white robes. It was my statue, and that was God Himself. Soon after our eyes met and his hands stopped. He looked at me with utmost love, with His powerful *drishti*. He came near me, caressed my hair and said, "I want to make your statue more beautiful and for that, I'll continue my work tomorrow." He blessed me and moved away.

I woke up with a jerk and found myself in my bed — back to this corporeal world in my own body **(Fig1.1)**. The moment I opened my eyes I felt some wetness and saw a red spot on the sheets. Spotting! Cancer? That was my first thought. I had seen many uterine cancer patients during my gynaecological practice for forty years but never thought that it could happen to me, especially because there was no family history of any type of cancer. At the age of 58, i.e. almost after 15 years of menopause, my story of the battle with cancer begins.

I decided to write a book on my healing journey the day my cancer diagnosis was confirmed. That same day, I started logging my daily trysts with the treatment and feelings.

This is the sixth year when I am writing my learnings from the divine healing

This book uncovers the diagnosis, my healing journey, the treatment I underwent, follow-up dilemma, emotional journey, learnings from my disease, tools and methods I used for healing and general precautions to take. It also elaborates preventive strategies for any type of female cancer. These learnings are beneficial not only for cancer fighters but also for other women and medical practitioners.

Healing Journey. What next?

The premonitory dream and my deductive reasoning were good enough reasons for me to consult my fellow gynaecologist. So, I called her up and the great friend she is, she asked me to immediately get investigated. The very next day, she examined me, made a pap smear and took an endometrial biopsy (a piece of the inner lining of the uterus).

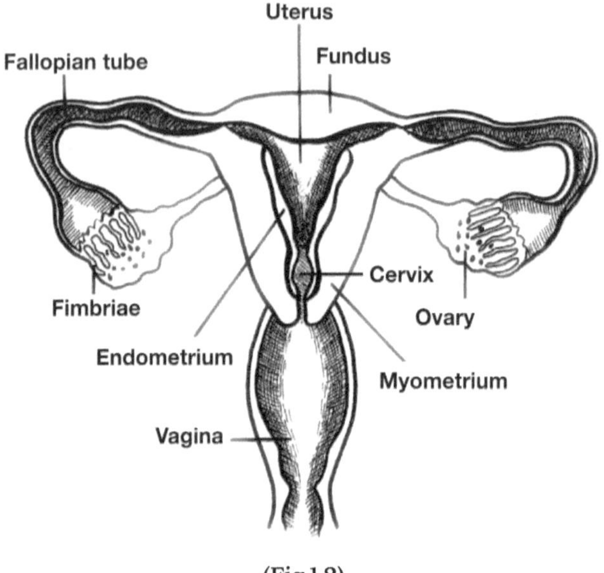

(Fig 1.2)

The test results showed some abnormal behaviour. The Pap test (conventional and LBC*) showed mild abnormal (dysplastic) changes. (Note: mild dysplasia report often comes +ve in an infection.)

So, I got my sonography done. Routinely, two tests are advised for someone who has post-menopausal spotting. The first test ultrasound showed 3mm endometrium (innermost linings of the uterus) uterus and the ovaries were normal. This report is deemed normal for a 58-year-old and 15 years post-menopausal woman (i.e. 3-5mm is the normal range). I thought that everything was fine.

But the second test advised was a biopsy of the inner lining of the uterus (endometrial biopsy). The report that came after a week showed abnormal patterns (few atypical endometrial).

The bleeding continued even after the biopsy. So I requested one of my seniors, a gynaecologist, for a hysterectomy, a surgery to remove the uterus.

Treatment dilemma-

I got my uterus removed (hysterectomy) by two divine senior doctors on 24 March 2017. Both the ovaries and the uterus were removed and sent for a biopsy. Although I was well after the surgery, a week later, the biopsy result came out as 'well-differentiated carcinoma'. The reports confirmed cancer of the uterus. Why did it happen to me? There was no family history of cancer! But I finally understood why God's hands had stopped abruptly in my dream.

Now the dilemma starts.

I consulted many onco-gynae surgeons and radiation oncologists from different institutes. Their advice varied. Few recommended a re-surgery (to remove the lymph nodes). However, most of them suggested waiting and following up in three months. Situational optimism crept in and I chose to wait.

After about a month, I had vertigo. I could not walk without support. So I visited a neuro physician. To rule out secondaries and find if cancer had spread, I got a CT scan of my brain done. Sigh of relief! No secondaries. The symptoms of vertigo were relieved within a month.

Recurrence

After three months of wait-and-see, I got a PET scan (scan of the whole body) and LBC (*liquid-based cytology advanced method of pap cytology) done. Both came normal. Nevertheless, the doctor was suspicious as she could not see the upper part (vault) of the lower genital tract (vagina) in the reports. Upon examination under anaesthesia, she found a slight bulge at the upper vault. It started bleeding the moment she touched it. The final PAP test indicated poorly differentiated vaginal epithelial cells recurrence. Whoops! Re-investigations.

I got my urinary bladder checked because I had blood in my urine a few times a couple of years back. Cystoscopy and vaginoscopy (examination of bladder and vagina by an endoscope) were done. The bladder was normal. However, the upper two-thirds of the lower genital tract (i.e. vagina) was filled with papillary growths. The biopsy taken from the growths showed an increased grade of cancer, adenocarcinoma with focal squamous differentiation.

Just as I had started to get comfortable, recurrence was confirmed after 5 months of hysterectomy. Endometrial carcinoma had spread to the vagina. Radiation along with adjuvant chemotherapy was the only way out. A CT scan showed no evidence of other abnormalities. Thankfully, it had not spread to other parts of the abdomen. Because two-thirds of the vagina was involved, the efficacy of radiation was not determinant.

Big decision and bigger dilemma! Big or a small Indian city for the treatment. When life gives you a dilemma, make dilemma-nade and have faith. Because I have complete faith in my fellow doctors and the state government medical facilities, I opted to get treated in my hometown. And so the radiation treatment, complete external and local brachytherapy, began.

Follow up dilemma

Radiation continued for 6 weeks. The follow-up pap smear showed moderately dysplastic epithelial cells along with radiation nucleomegaly. I had to get tested every three months the following year. Unexpectedly, the reports kept showing the same abnormal pattern. To top that off, I had also developed many radiation side-effects like proctitis, loss of appetite, black stool, nausea and weakness.

Another dilemma-nade opportunity! Since the reports were not showing much progress, I decided to use the healing power of meditation. I continued taking the daily meditation pill. God's hands had started taking care of me. After a year and a half of spiritual healing, the reports came out normal finally. Although, some side effects like proctitis lingered for almost two years.

Emotional wellbeing: Diagnosis, and recurrence-

Most patients when diagnosed with cancer go through different emotional stages.

Shock: This phase may range from complete denial to just acting as if nothing is wrong.

Fear: People are worried that they are going to die.

Guilt: People may blame themselves for past choices that could be related to the diagnosis or feel guilt for burdening loved ones.

Loss: A person's sense of self can be taken over by cancer and treatments.

Acceptance: Slowly and gradually, people adapt and move forward.

My emotions during the diagnosis

I had been practising meditation for almost 35 years. There was no family history of cancer whatsoever. Also, it's a known fact that 90% of postmenopausal bleeding is benign. With this pretext, I was in denial since the first spotting.

Acceptance

When the report showed 'cancer', I accepted it and was ready for future consequences. I surrendered everything to God and started using my spiritual knowledge learned at the Brahma Kumaris Vishwa Vidyalaya, a spiritual organization based in Mount Abu, India.

These spiritual practices helped me get into the acceptance phase from the denial phase very easily. I was emotionally stable. I did not have to pass the stages that most cancer patients felt emotionally.

Just seven days after the surgery, I was giving a meditation course to a patient suffering from depression. When the biopsy report was handed over to me, I perused the report myself before informing my husband about the cancer diagnosis. I was in a peaceful mental state. I was happy and emotionally stable the entire time. Whenever someone would ask about my health, I would tell them that even though I was diagnosed with uterine cancer, it is 'well differentiated' and that I will be well soon.

My emotions during recurrence-

A little string of doubt had indeed crept in after recurrence when it became 'poorly differentiated'. That is when I recalled a positive verse from the daily teachings of the Brahma Kumaris:

"When you change the negative to positive, the world will change".

I felt that I should be an example to society and take this as a challenge. So I started focusing more on spiritual practices. I practised the healing power of affirmations, visualisation and meditation, and took no treatment after the radiation. Ever since, every year, I follow up with a pap smear and pelvic USG. And now the reports are normal, I am fine and more energetic than ever.

I had prayed to God to not let cancer disturb my spiritual and other services. The inflammatory effects of radiation and chemotherapy had caused a loss of appetite, proctitis (inflammation of the rectum) and weakness, but luckily I did not lose my hair and cancer did not show in my appearance. Every day I used to drive to the radiation department myself and never missed seeing my patients.

Over the weekends, I travelled alone by train for Godly service in other cities. The Supreme surgeon and the blessings of my divine family and patients helped me heal and kept me stable.

Just as I finished writing this first chapter, I got a call for another case of endometrial biopsy which reminded me of my case. During the patient's biopsy procedure cheesy endometrium had come out, which was suspicious of cancer. The incidence of endometrial cancer is increasing in India. That is when I realised that I should complete this book ASAP for awareness.

My healing journey reminds me of this quote from the famous writer, Maya Angelou:

"Still, when it looked like the sun wasn't going to shine anymore, God put a rainbow in the clouds".

Summary

- With recent medical advancements and a positive mental status, healing is easier than ever. A positive attitude helps prevent treatment side-effects from meddling with your life.
- Be powerful. Spread positivity around you and inspire society.

- Spirituality helps to keep the mind stable and positive throughout the journey.

Chapter 2

New lessons I Learned

"Life is not a holiday but an education.
And the one eternal question for us all is how better
we can love."

-Henry Drummond

Life is a beautiful journey filled with many obstacles. While overcoming these life hurdles we often make mistakes. With a growth mindset, we can learn from these mistakes and share our experiences with others.

"Learn from the mistakes of others. You can't live
long enough to make them all yourself."

-Eleanor Roosevelt

I have always considered my mistakes as my teacher. This has indeed made my life journey divine and healthy. I am sharing my learnings intending to benefit you. Later, I also touched upon some of the great opportunities I got during my healing journey.

First, I will pen down the mistakes I made a few years before and after getting the disease-

- I used to suppress my feelings which may have been one of the triggers of the disease
- I ignored the signals that my body gave during the perimenopausal period (around 40 years of age)
- I did not follow a proper guideline for managing the disease

First mistake: The psychological- I suppressed my feelings for a long time

We often suppress our feelings when dealing with adverse situations or difficult people. It leads to repressed anger and chronic stress which could grow into cancer later on in life. It is hard to perceive the effects of suppression in a short time.

Now you would ask, how can chronic emotional stress cause cancer?

Stress suppresses the immune system. Elevated stress hormone increases glucose levels within normal cells. Pathogenic microbes (virus, bacteria, fungus) attack normal cells to feed on the glucose. This leads to a lack of oxygen and reduced cell energy. Eventually, normal cells start to mutate and create new cancer cells. The microbes use cancer cells as hosts and stimulate cells to propagate even more, eventually transforming into a tumour.

After all, what is suppression?

Emotional suppression is inhibiting the outward signs of your inner feelings. It is often a negative feeling against someone. The subject experiencing it does not express their feelings. Initially, they don't desire to see or communicate with that person. Gradually, they develop a hatred for them.

Let's understand this by an example. Say, we have a mother-in-law (M-I-L) and daughter-in-law (D-I-L) duo. Both have some expectations from each other. With time, the M-I-L starts criticising the D-I-L because she does not fulfil her expectations. The D-I-L, however, is unable to express her feelings. So she suppresses them. This suppression is similar to the pressure built up in a pressure cooker which could burst at any moment.

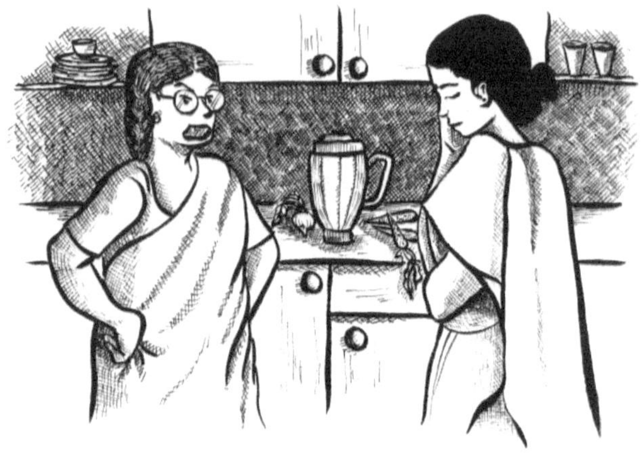

(Fig 2.1)

In the year 1990, I had to move to a new city to live with my joint family. I had been an independent woman until then, albeit a very shy one. I would not utter a word when things didn't happen as I wanted or when I was unnecessarily reprimanded. However, I would feel miserable after every such incident. One of my family members was irrationally arrogant to almost everyone, especially me. I could not speak up, so it kept bottling up for a few years. To add to the build-up, back at the hospital, I was assigned to a department that I didn't like. I am certain that all of this was the germination of the slow-growing endometrial cancer in me.

I am sharing this experience so that you are aware of the harmful effects of emotional suppression. I hope to convince you to change your attitude if you feel you have been taciturn like I was.

Lessons learned from the first mistake

First lesson- I am sure you would have guessed by now that we should never suppress our feelings. We should rather be **assertive,** which is basically putting forth our views with composure. **Being assertive implies not being aggressive and reactive, even when someone is angry. They could be wrong at the time, but assertiveness says to put your views in front of them after they have cooled down. (Fig 2.2).**

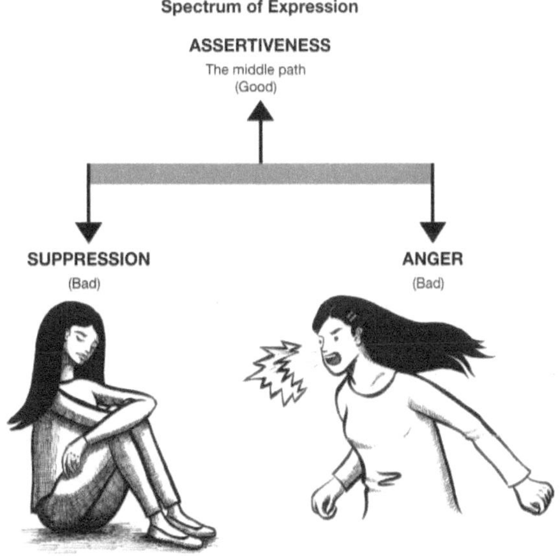

Fig 2.2

The second lesson learned- This world is a drama and we are playing our parts

All the world's a stage,

And all the men and women merely players;

They have their exits and their entrances;

-William Shakespeare

Have you ever seen actors in their real lives ever getting offended by a villain's bad behaviour in a drama? In fact, a bad role, if acted well, is commended. Similarly, we play our parts in this world drama. The bad behaviours of our co-actors should not impact us. We must accept everyone as they are.

Imagine yourself to be a hero of this drama and believe you have the power to change every negative into a positive. There is always more than one way to see anything, so allow yourself to see only the positive, hopeful and cheerful aspects of life.

Third lesson- Another important lesson I learned was that life is too short to suppress your emotions. If someone insults you, ignore it, simple! This reminds me of a story -

A woman climbed up a bus and took a seat beside a man, intentionally hitting him with her numerous bags. But the man remained silent. The curious woman asked him why he did not complain when her bags hit him?

The man replied with a smile:

"There is no need to be upset about something so insignificant, our journey together is very short, because I'm getting off at the next stop."

The woman apologized and excused herself.

We must understand that our time in this world is so short that darkening it with useless arguments, jealousy, unforgivenness, discontentment and bad attitude is a ridiculous waste of time and energy.

Did someone break your heart? Stay calm. The trip is too short.

Did someone betray, intimidate, cheat or humiliate you? Relax - Don't Be Stressed. The trip is too short.

Did someone insult you without a reason? Stay calm. Ignore it. The trip is too short.

Did someone make a comment that you didn't like? Stay calm. Ignore. Forgive, keep them in your prayers and love them still for no reason. The trip is too short.

Whatever the problem falls upon us, it is a problem if we think of it as a problem! Remember, our journey together is too short.

No one knows the length of their trip. No one has seen tomorrow. Nobody knows when it will arrive at its stop.

Fourth lesson- There is more to the list of significant lessons learned like how to transform suppression into tolerance power. Tolerance is a virtue and suppression is a negative feeling. I bet those years taught me valuable life lessons which made me stronger. Even though I had been practising spirituality, I could not apply them practically. After those few years of learning, I understood that by accepting everyone as they are, much of our wasted energy can be saved. I also learned how to deal with tough people. Neither do I have any guilt for my past mistakes nor do I blame anyone. But, I sure have learned from my past. As I started accepting everyone's behaviour my tolerance power automatically increased.

Second big mistake: The physical- I ignored signals from my body

In the fast-paced world we are always so busy in our routines that we do not have time to take care of ourselves. This story of a seven-year-old depicts how much we are caught up in our lives, that we even forget to notice important things around us.

A seven-year-old boy was trying to stop every car that passed by a busy street. He was waving his

hands vigorously to get some attention, but no one stopped, no one even noticed. This continued for a few hours. Eventually, the exhausted kid picked up a stone and hit the next car that went by. In the car was a famous businessman. The car stopped and out came the businessman grumbling, "Who the hell has damaged my car?"

The gentleman started scolding the boy. The scared boy pointed his finger to the side to draw his attention. The businessman saw that a crying two-year-old had fallen from the wheelchair. The boy said, "Sir, I am sorry but I could not help my brother and have been trying to get help for the last three hours." The businessman stopped grumbling and his eyes welled up with tears. He helped his brother sit back in the wheelchair.

And you know what! The businessman never fixed the dent that the stone had left.

Why? Because in this busy life sometimes we ignore many important things. God sends us signals to take care of our health but often, err! mostly, we ignore it. He then throws some stones at us in the form of the disease so that we take out some time for ourselves.

Lesson learned from second mistake

The fifth lesson- Listen to your body and prioritize health. I ignored irregular bleeding during perimenopause, i.e. before the cessation of menses around 40-45 years. Our body sends us signals that we often overlook. I had menorrhagia, excessive menstrual bleeding, during perimenopause in my forties. So I got a D&C done. It is a short procedure in which an inside piece of the uterine lining is sent for biopsy. My biopsy report was abnormal (endometrial hyperplasia with few atypical patterns). In medical terms, it is an abnormal pattern with endometrial gland proliferation. I took hormonal treatment (progesterone) for 6 months. Menstruation stopped and so I did not follow up further. There is a 10% chance that this abnormal endometrium may turn malignant in a few years. After 15 years of menopause, when I developed cancer, I realized my mistake that I should have followed up after menstruation had stopped. Now, I always advise my patients,

"Don't ignore excessive, prolonged or irregular bleeding during perimenopause. Don't be too busy with your routine, give health a priority. Consult your gynaecologist, get a USG and endometrial biopsy done!"

Endometrial cancer is an increasing trend worldwide. A regular follow up with your doctor is necessary if atypical abnormal endometrial hyperplasia is detected. Do not ignore it like me!

What is normal menopause?

Menopause refers to the end of the menstrual cycle. Twelve months without any period indicates that you have hit menopause. The time before menopause is called perimenopause. In normal menopause, menses suddenly stops or you get scanty menses i.e. every 2-3 months. Heavy bleeding is not normal. Bleeding after a year of menopause is called postmenopausal bleeding.

Third mistake- I did not follow proper protocol for diagnosing the disease myself

Lesson learned from the third mistake-

Sixth Lesson- A methodical approach is necessary to cure any disease.

Just as I started writing this part, a doctor dropped by to show his wife's sonography report. Transvaginal sonography showed an abnormal inner lining of the uterus (endometrial hyperplasia). He inquired if they could get the uterus removed. This is the most common mistake that most patients, even medical doctors make. I shared my cancer story with him, "I had postmenopausal bleeding, my pap smear and sonography were normal. The only abnormality was slightly abnormal atypical hyperplasia in the biopsy. However, I directly got my hysterectomy done without going for further investigations." Diagnosis of carcinoma after surgery confuses the treatment. I further said, "I learned that even a little abnormality in any test or investigation should not be ignored. Hysteroscopy is a diagnostic endoscopic procedure that makes visualization of the uterus possible. It is the 'Gold standard' for diagnosing endometrial carcinoma." After listening to my story, the doctor was convinced to further investigate.

I had never thought that I could get cancer because there was no family history, I was wrong. Anyone can get this drastic disease, be aware of it and be vigilant.

A patient once came to me with her abnormal sonography report of endometrial hyperplasia. She had heavy bleeding. I advised her for a biopsy. A biopsy is necessary if endometrial hyperplasia is detected in sonography at around 40 years of age. In India, ignorance about malignancy is very high. People assume that irregular bleeding is normal. Even this patient did not understand the gravity of the matter. She was reluctant to get the procedure done, rather she wanted to get it fixed with medicines.

I recall another incident from about five years ago when a patient in the advanced stages of carcinoma in the cervix came to me for consultation. I had referred her to the radiation department for radiation therapy, but she assumed that she would be cured by hysterectomy alone, and eventually only got the uterus removed. A year later her relatives informed me about her demise. A step-by-step procedure is necessary for the investigation and treatment of any disease.

The opportunities I got during my healing disease

This second part of the chapter describes how the disease presented a twist and gave a new dimension to my life. It is said that every cloud has a silver lining. Every situation gives us a unique opportunity to progress in our lives.

"However, aside from work, I have little joy. In the end, wealth is only a fact of life that I am accustomed to. Material things lost can be found. But there is one thing that can never be found when it is lost – 'Life'. Whichever stage in life we are at right now, with time, we will face the day when the curtain comes down. Treasure Love for your family, love for your spouse, love for your friends... Treat yourself well. Cherish others."

-Steve Jobs

First opportunity- The first and most important opportunity that cancer presented to me was to serve cancer patients and others who fear cancer.

Typically, when cancer is diagnosed questions like these may arise in our minds:

- Why me?
- What will happen in the future?
- Has God punished me?
- How can I remain stable, enthusiastic and enjoy the journey of life even in adverse circumstances?
- How can I forget the past?

Surprisingly, most of the healthy people with a family history of cancer live in a fear of developing it, which does no good. So, along with cancer patients, I started taking sessions for the general public on awareness and prevention of cancer and its recurrence in the long term. In these sessions, I cover answers to the questions listed above, my experiences and the healing tools I used, all of which are covered in the second section of this book.

Second opportunity- The **second opportunity** was to serve the medical fraternity. I sometimes participate in various medical workshops and speak on how positivity helps in healing. Some common emotions that the patients, their families, and friends experience when they first hear about the diagnosis are shock, fear, sadness, depression, and guilt. It is a common experience that anyone who has a positive mindset has a healing touch. To begin with, patients should share their diagnosis with such a person. Even doctors should inform about the cancer diagnosis to a person with a positive mindset from the patient's family or friends. In my case, I was the first to know that I was diagnosed with cancer. Indeed, I was surprised, but I did not have any negative emotions because of my meditative lifestyle.

Third opportunity- The next opportunity I got was to explore spiritual knowledge deeper. Spirituality reminds us of our life's purpose. I explored my purpose and spiritual knowledge while performing each ***karma*** and I felt as if God, the 'Supreme Surgeon', was always beside me, taking care of me.

There is a common misconception about the meaning of 'purpose of life'. In a true sense, your purpose should answer the question, "Why am I here?". We will dive into it in the second section.

Fourth opportunity- Finally, the opportunity to write down my experiences in a book. I wrote this book because I had promised the Supreme Surgeon that I would write a book on my cancer healing journey after 5 years of diagnosis. This was the best opportunity I got. I am thankful to God that he made me His instrument to serve society.

"Turn your wounds into wisdom"

- Oprah Winfrey

Summary

- Chronic stress (suppression) leads to cancer. Never suppress your feelings, change your attitude and be assertive.
- Give your health a priority, don't ignore signals given by the body.
- Be vigilant and cautious if biopsy reports suggest atypical hyperplasia (abnormal).
- A step-by-step procedure should be followed in the diagnosis and treatment of any disease.
- Never feel guilt from mistakes of the past. Share your experiences and make everyone blessed.

Section 2

Tools for my Healing

"Healing is a choice. It's not an easy one because it takes work to turn around your habits. But keep making the choice and shifts will happen."

— Yehuda Berg

The term healing is derived from the word 'heal' which means to make something whole again. It is a holistic and transformative process of repair and recovery of the mind, body and spirit. It brings about a positive change in the healed. Regardless of the presence or absence of any disease, the healing process, in fact, is finding meaning and movement towards self-realization of wholeness.

Modern medicine does not train today's physicians to be true healers. I consider myself lucky to have learned both modern medicine and spirituality, the healing tool. Both are necessary for treating diseases and healing the mind and body. These tools have sided with me throughout my healing journey. Indeed, my spiritual practice since 1986 helped me overcome my fears and side effects of the treatment, however, it was during this time that I realized preaching is easier than practical application. I am grateful that my healing journey allowed me to hone my healing skills and made me more experienced. This section further elaborates on how to leverage the tools.

"Happiness is the best immunity booster"

Chapter 3

How to Build Physical Immunity

"No doctor has ever healed anyone of anything in the history of the world. The human immune system heals and that's the only thing that heals"

-Bob Wright

The Merriam Webster dictionary defines 'risk' as the possibility of loss or injury. A cancer risk factor is anything that increases the chance of getting cancer. The general risk factors for cancer are mainly lifestyle, exposure to noxious substances, hormone imbalance and heredity. Particularly, a high body mass index (aka. BMI is a measure of body fat based on height and weight), a low intake of fruits and vegetables, lack of physical activity, the use of alcohol and smoking are the five most pronounced risk factors in the onset of several types of cancers. Some chronic infections like the Human Papilloma Virus (HPV) may lead to genital (or cervical) cancer.

Some of these risk factors can be avoided by simple lifestyle changes, the most crucial being an active lifestyle, a healthy diet and proper sleep. These are not only important to prevent cancer but also to heal and keep healthy holistically.

Holistic health is a widely talked about concept these days. It is an approach to life that considers multi-dimensional aspects of wellness. It encourages us to keep our bodies physically, emotionally and spiritually healthy. All three aspects are necessary to build immunity and I was determined to heal myself holistically.

Physical immunity

The immune system is a complex network of biological processes that defends our bodies against harmful microorganisms and infections. Everyone is born with innate immunity. We should maintain it or else it wanes with time.

There are two aspects to immunity - physical and emotional

Physical immunity protects us from infections from the environment. A healthy lifestyle, good diet, exercise, proper sleep and taking essential medicine boost physical immunity. These habits help maintain good body weight and prevent extra fat deposition in the body, thus, normalizing the blood glucose level. Essential medicine and vitamins are also necessary to prevent infections and increase immunity during the treatment.

In the initial phases of my healing journey, I had started to explore physical healing. I soon realized that to heal myself I needed to maintain a good body weight, a healthy lifestyle, a good diet and a regular exercise regime.

Weight reduction

W.H.O. defines obesity and overweight as abnormal or excessive fat accumulation that may impair health. Obesity is one of the most common causes of non-infectious diseases like diabetes, hypertension and cancer. People who have less muscle mass and comparatively excessive fat are more prone to cancer.

Waist size is considered a good indicator of health. A large waist circumference indicates excessive abdominal fat. Research indicates that risk goes up with a waist size that is greater than 35 inches for women or greater than 40 inches for men.

The modern advancements and job requirements have resulted in a more sedentary lifestyle. In a sedentary lifestyle, there is little to no physical activity. It is a dangerous trend of this century. 39% of adults are obese worldwide. Stress, overeating, sedentary lifestyle, hormonal imbalance and an increased reliance on medicine are some of the other causes of obesity.

The body mass index (BMI) is used as a screening tool for determining overweight and obesity. BMI over 25 is considered overweight, and over 30 is obese.

<u>Formula</u>: BMI = wt in kg / (height in meter)^2

Excessive weight and obesity present an 11% increased risk of cancer in women. There are 13 types of cancers associated with obesity; uterine and colorectal breast cancers to name a few. Visceral organs are the soft internal organs of the body including the lungs, the heart, and the organs of the digestive, excretory, reproductive, and circulatory systems. Excess visceral fats cause inflammation and increased insulin and oestrogen hormone levels which can cause cancers such as endometrial hyperplasia, endometrial cancer, ovarian cancer and postmenopausal breast cancer.

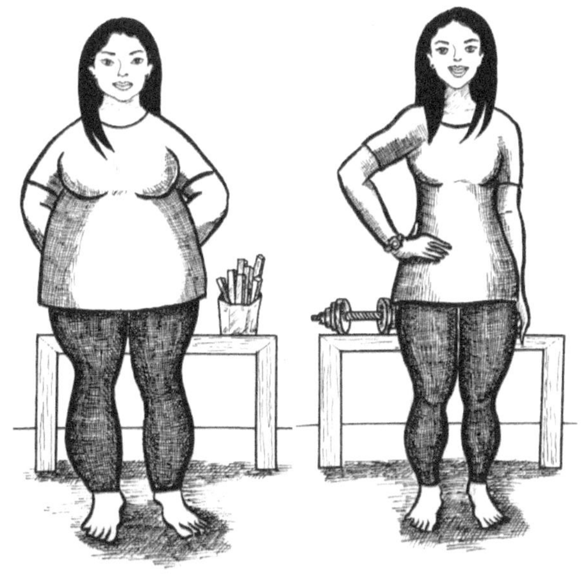

(Fig 3.1)

Although I've never looked fat, my muscle mass was less compared to my body's fat percentage. I was not doing enough exercise to maintain a good balance of both. At this stage, I realised that even if you do not appear fat but the muscle mass is less, you are still prone to the disease and these imbalances may lead to endometrial abnormalities. Diabetes is also considered a risk factor for cancer. I was a borderline diabetic, my blood sugar level would sometimes show as raised. Normal blood sugar is between 90-110 mg when fasting, and 120-140 mg post-meal.

Immunity-Boosting Diet

"You are what you eat."

Diet is food or drinks regularly consumed by an individual. Dieting is regulating your diet to improve your physical condition. I was overwhelmed by the variety of diet plans I found during my physical healing research. Some diet plans had a high protein content, some recommended low protein intake while some vouched for fasting. Some suggested a mono-diet while some others recommended consuming multi-coloured food. This diet planning conundrum reminds me of a brilliant short story I recently heard.

Once a group of five friends, out on an excursion, lost their way back from a dense forest. When they reached the crossroads, they were confused and wanted to take different paths.

The first friend exclaimed, "I am going left."

The second friend disagreed and said, "I'd rather take the right.

The third was sceptical of taking new routes and said, "I know the way back is arduous, but I am going to retrace our footsteps."

The fourth one had always wanted to be a pioneer and expressed, "I want to forge a new path."

The fifth friend, thinking that others were foolish, climbed a tree and shouted, "I see a village close by, I am going to seek their help."

Who of the five friends was right?

All of them. Let us see what happened to each of them on their individual paths. The first friend did not get any food. He learned the art of fasting and so increased his inner power. He came out more experienced than ever. The second friend increased his tolerance power and became stronger by fighting bandits who attacked him. The third one safely reached the campsite and found people who helped him get back. The fourth one created new possibilities for others. The fifth one found a shortcut but he too was right to seek help.

Similarly, all theories and researches are probably right. We should adopt the one that suits us best, of course, backed up by our own intuition and research.

Eventually, with some more research and consultation, I adopted a plan suitable for vegetarians.

According to the American Institute for Cancer Research's (AICR) Guidelines for Cancer Survivors, vegetarian diets seem to confer protection against cancer. You can reduce your cancer risk by choosing a variety of vegetables, fruits, beans and whole grains while limiting red meat. Human anatomy and physiology also reveal that a human being is basically vegetarian. Like herbivores (plant-eating animals), our large and small intestines measure four times the length of our body, whereas, for carnivores (meat-eating animals), it is approximately the same size. Moreover, we do not have fangs like the carnivores who have to bite the flesh. Human saliva is alkaline and contains ptyalin to digest carbohydrates, whereas, in carnivores, it is acidic. For carnivores to digest a highly proteinaceous flesh diet, gastric secretions in the stomach are highly acidic, whereas the human secretion has lower acidity.

A vegetarian diet does not give 100% protection from cancer. The various pesticides and chemicals used in farming are toxic and carcinogenic. However, we can take control of what is in our hands.

I had to change my dietary pattern during the treatment. Initially, during radiotherapy, because I could not digest a high protein diet, I had to stop taking pulses that are high in protein. I observed that raw foods were digestible and comfortable. Consuming raw food is healthy. Uncooked food is close to nature and makes the medium alkaline which prevents many infections. Cooked food is acidic in nature and not good for the body.

Raw Turmeric

One of my doctor friends had suggested trying raw turmeric during my treatment. Raw turmeric contains curcumin which has shown great benefits in cancer treatment. It also helps chemotherapy work better. It has been seen that cancer occurrences are less in countries where people eat more curcumin. Fresh raw turmeric also increases our immunity. Turmeric is antioxidant, antiviral and antifungal, and helps in the growth of healthy bacteria.

Every morning I slowly drink a glass of boiled water with grated raw turmeric, ginger and a little black pepper. Absorption of turmeric increases 2000 fold when consumed with black pepper. I also add raw turmeric to my salads. To wrap my day I have half a cup of turmeric milk.

After seeing the benefits first-hand, I started growing turmeric in my home. I now advise my patients complaining about leucorrhoea to consume raw turmeric. Leucorrhoea is a thick, whitish, yellowish or greenish vaginal discharge that is mainly experienced during puberty when sexual organs are developing in a woman. The antiseptic properties of turmeric ease the symptoms.

Fruits and vegetables

The American Cancer Society recommend five servings of fruits and vegetables a day. During radiation therapy, my intestines were inflamed and so I could not eat much. I would consume very small portions of multi-coloured fruits, vegetables, fresh fruit juice and coconut water 3-4 times every day. After radiation, I started taking full portions of fruits and vegetables for both breakfast and lunch. Multi-coloured fruits are nutritious and also maintain a healthy weight. Tomatoes contain lycopene, the pigment which gives normal red colour which reduces the risk of several types of cancer. Fruits and vegetables should be washed with soda-bicarbonate mixed water which has been found to reduce the effect of pesticides.

Bhagavad Gita describes raw fruits and vegetables as a *satwik* diet.

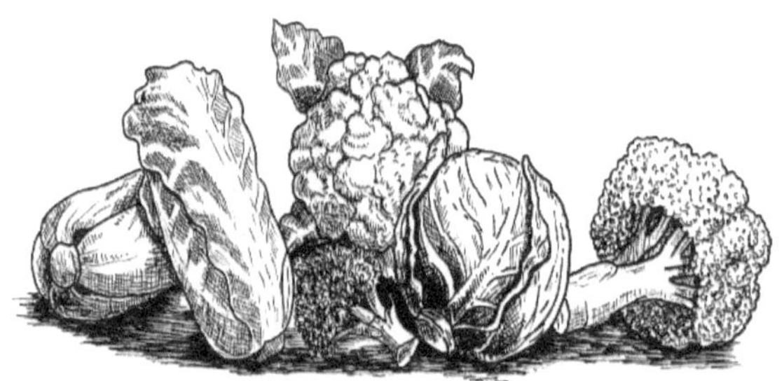

(Fig 3.2)

I increased certain fruits and vegetables that are said to have anti-cancer properties like the cabbage family- cruciferous vegetables, broccoli, cauliflower and brussels sprouts.

A high intake of products rich in fibre (e.g. whole grains), flax seeds that contain omega-3 fatty acids and a moderate intake of milk and dairy may reduce the incidence of different types of cancer.

Many essential vitamins are present in fruits and vegetables, which are also necessary for healing. Vitamin-A can be found in carrot, mango and papaya, Vitamin-B in green leafy vegetables, fenugreek, palak, sprouted grain and Vitamin-C in citrous fruit, lemon, orange, amla. Vitamin D can be increased by daily sunbathing for 15-20 minutes.

Water and other fluids

I consume about 6-8 glasses of liquid every day. It lowers the concentration of potential cancer-causing agents. By drinking "charged water" in the morning anyone can detoxify their digestive system. To prepare charged water, hold the glass of water and visualize positive thoughts and affirmations for as long as you want.

Before consuming, I offer my food and water to God **(Fig 3.3)**. I then give healing vibrations to it. That is not all, while drinking and eating I visualise that it is my medicine and my body is being healed. It is not possible to completely remove pesticides and the negativity that gets absorbed from the negative stressful environment of present times, from food. There are many studies that prove the effect of thoughts on water and food which we will discuss in the next chapter.

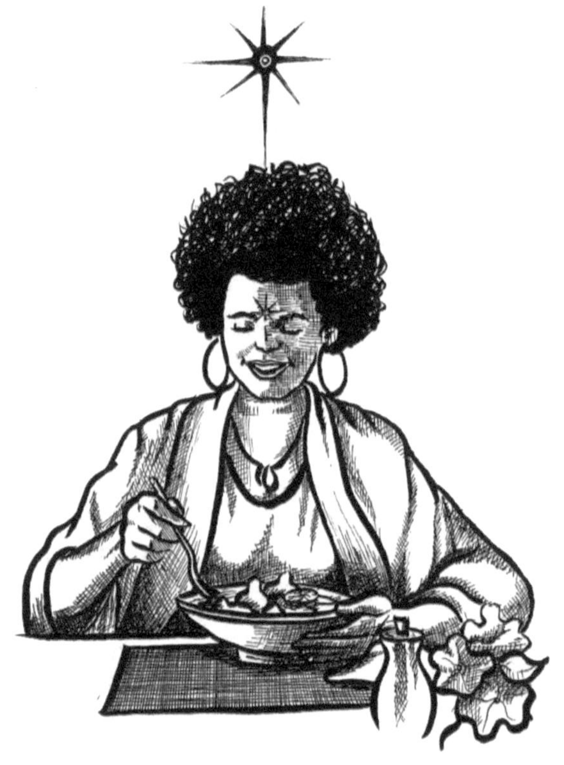

(Fig 3.3)

The Mediterranean diet is considered one of the healthiest dietary patterns. It is a combination of foods rich mainly in antioxidants and anti-inflammatory nutrients. Many studies have demonstrated a strong and inverse relationship between a high level of Mediterranean diet, adherence and some chronic diseases (such as cardiovascular diseases, diabetes, etc.) and cancer. Given its protective effects in reducing oxidative and inflammatory processes of cells and avoiding DNA damages, cell proliferation, and their survival, angiogenesis, inflammations and metastasis, the Mediterranean diet is considered a powerful and manageable method to fight cancer incidence. The Mediterranean diet varies by country and region, so it has a range of definitions. But in general, it is high in vegetables, fruits, legumes, nuts, beans, cereals, grains, fish, and unsaturated fats such as olive oil. It usually includes a low intake of dairy foods, meat and animal products. Animal fats and oils, often cooked at high temperatures, may increase cancer incidence.

Things I avoided

Early on I had the habit of having morning tea or chai. I quit chai during the radiation therapy. And there began the path to becoming a perfect Yogi. I have heard of a real story about a tea enthusiastic yogi on his deathbed. In his last moments, when he was offered food (i.e. *bhog/prasad*), instead of accepting it with love and thankfulness, he kept searching for tea. In the Bhagavad Gita God says, "Whoever at the time of death, quits his body, remembering Me alone, at once attains My nature."

I also limited the frequency of cooked and fried food. It produces harmful chemical compounds. I adopted steamed or baked food. Steaming and baking both increase the bioavailability and decrease the formation of harmful compounds.

I also avoided junk food like *maida*, excess salt, stale and excess food.

Physical activity and Exercise

Any type of activity that uses skeletal muscles and requires more energy than resting is beneficial. Research shows that exercise is safe, improves the quality of life and increases energy in cancer survivors. Physical activity may also help cope with the side effects of the treatment and possibly decrease the risk of new cancers in future. Exercise for cancer survivors can also keep cancer from recurring. 150 minutes of moderate activity or 75 minutes of vigorous activity each week is recommended by the American cancer society for cancer prevention and recurrence. Strength training exercise at least two days each week is necessary for cancer survivors.

Start slow and build up as per your capacity. Although I was exercising before the diagnosis, I was not a regular. During my radiation treatment, it was not possible for me to exercise so I only performed routine household work and examined a few outdoor patients. After finishing radiation therapy I started yogic walking every day for half an hour. In a yogic stroll, you visualise that sun rays are emanating from God and falling upon you to purify you. You also thank God for the gift of life. Some days I would do fat burning group exercises. Group exercises boost motivation and make exercising fun.

An active healthy lifestyle helps not only in cancer prevention but also is good for cancer survivors. How does regular exercising benefit before, during, and after cancer treatment?

- Reduces inflammation
- Maintains blood sugar
- Maintains or improves physical ability to get things done
- Lowering sex hormones such as estrogen, prevents the high levels of insulin which are linked to cancer development
- Improves mood

- Reduces depression and anxiety
- Boosts self-confidence and helps your body and brain work better
- Reduces fatigue
- Increases immunity power and controls weight
- Might help sleep better
- Increases appetite
- Decreases the chances of some types of cancer recurrence
- Improves quality of life
- During chemotherapy exercise can help ease side effects, such as fatigue and nausea, and can help boost your immune system

Types of Exercises

Exercise needs to vary with individuals. We don't yet know the best amount and level of exercise for someone with cancer. The goal of my exercise program during my treatment was to keep up my muscle strength and maintain my ability to perform daily activities. I exercised in the mornings and combined different types to keep it fun and complete.

Stretching is a subtle exercise that everyone can do. It is important to keep moving and keep the body flexible and balanced.

Aerobic exercises, such as brisk walking, jogging and swimming, helps you lose weight. I chose walking. This type of exercise burns calories. An exercise program consisting of half an hour of aerobic exercise three times a week is sufficient to improve anxiety, depression, fatigue, quality of life and physical function in cancer survivors.

Pranayam or breath control also helps reduce stress and improves mental clarity. In particular, a study published in BMC Complementary and Alternative Medicine Therapies found that stress-related markers in saliva were decreased with only 20-minutes of yoga breathing.

Resistance training is a form of exercise that improves muscle strength and endurance. Some kind of resistance training like weightlifting, resistance bands etc. are necessary at least twice a week.

Sleep Management

Good quality of sleep is very important in the healing and prevention of any disease. Sleep deprivation is one of the causes of diseases. Getting enough sleep is important for your health. For some people, just 5 hours of sleep is sufficient, whereas some others wake up tired even after 8 hours of sleep. In short, the quality of sleep is more important than its duration. Insomnia is when you have trouble falling or staying asleep at night. Because of my daily meditation practice, I was fortunate to not have any problems with my previous sleep pattern. Just for a few days during my brachytherapy treatment, I had increased vaginal itching at night. So, for 2-3 days I had to take mild sedatives and treatment for itching.

Healing occurs during sleep because melatonin produced by the brain during sleep may have antioxidant properties that help prevent damage to cells that can lead to cancer. In addition, melatonin lowers estrogen production from the ovaries. Thus, a lack of sleep leads to insufficient melatonin. This series of events may expose women to high levels of estrogen and may increase the risk of estrogen-dependent cancers.

It is common for patients to experience insomnia during and after treatment. If insomnia is not treated, it can add to the existing symptoms such as pain, fatigue and anxiety. Common causes of insomnia include:

- Stress, anxiety, or depression
- Physical discomforts, such as headaches, nausea, vomiting, hot flashes, or pain
- Side effects from medication, chemotherapy or radiation
- Conditions such as acid reflux, thyroid issues, or bladder problems

Unfamiliar environments or changes to routines, such as an overnight stay at the hospital

Because I practised morning meditation and listened to positive versions taught at the Brahma Kumaris, I did not feel any stress that cancer patients complain about. I always advise my patients to start their day with positive reading or positive listening. Some Research, including Spiegel's study, shows that cancer patients who manage their stress in group therapy, with good social networks, or with regular exercise often fare better than patients who don't manage stress effectively.

Most adults need approximately 7-8 hours of sleep every night to function at their best. However, for those who practice meditation only 5-6 hours of good quality sleep is sufficient. For good sleep, sleep hygiene is necessary.

Sleep hygiene

Good sleep hygiene is one of the best ways to prepare for better sleep. It is important for both physical and mental healing. A stable sleep schedule, healthy diet, regular exercise, the physical environment and regulated screen time all contribute to ideal sleep hygiene. The pre and post bed routines I follow have improved my overall well-being.

Pre-sleep habits help you fall asleep faster by decompressing and slowing down the brain. A giant key to getting up early is sleeping deeply. I sleep according to my biological clock, usually between 10 p.m. to 4 a.m. To prepare, I finish dinner by 8 p.m. and avoid eating heavy meals, spicy foods or sugary items close to bedtime. Light exposure from backlit electronic devices within four hours before natural sleep onset shifts our biological clocks and makes it harder to fall asleep. At night, I avoid all electronic devices as much as possible and keep them in a different room. Exercising close to bedtime makes you stimulated and energized and can move the sleep time later. Meditation, on the contrary, releases serotonin (the sleep hormone) and relaxes our mind and body. Every night before bed, I empty my mind and recall a positive memory from the day and express gratitude to those who have helped me (**Fig 3.4**), and end with half-an-hour meditation practice.

For a sound sleep, a post-bed routine is as important as a pre-bed routine. A well-structured routine will help the brain separate day from night better. I leave my bedroom right after waking up and then meditate for an hour. Morning exercise increases our energy levels, alertness and focus. I exercise in the mornings and take a 20-minute mid-afternoon restful nap. Napping has a lot of benefits like increased memory, improved job performance, reduced stress and so on. I completely removed caffeinated drinks from my diet. Research has shown that caffeine interferes with circadian melatonin rhythm and delays the onset of sleep if consumed close to bedtime. Green tea is believed to be a strong cancer fighter, organic decaffeinated Green tea and lemon combination has good protective effects. I often drink organic green tea in the evenings.

The ambience and physical setting of the bedroom are vital for getting a sound sleep. I keep my room cool, quiet and dark. My bedding is clean and comfortable. I wear loose clothing. The right sleepwear is important for a good night's sleep.

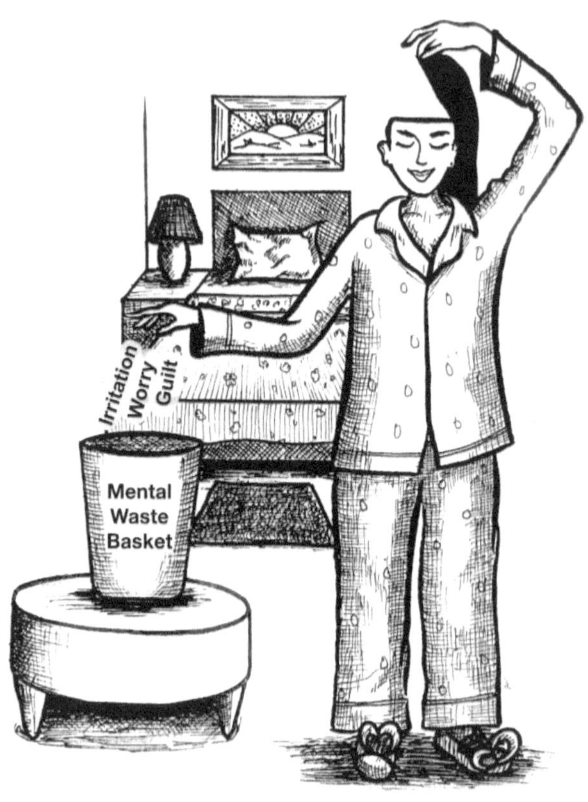

(Fig 3.4)

Summary

- Obesity is one of the causes of cancer. Weight reduction is very essential to avoid many types of cancer.
- A healthy diet that includes raw fruits and vegetables, and ample liquid is

required for the prevention of cancer and recommended for cancer survivors.

- Exercise is scientifically proven to prevent cancer and its recurrence.
- Sleeping according to the biological clock is necessary to keep hormonal balance and support healing.

Chapter 4

How I Boost My Emotional Immunity

"Even the smallest shift in perspective can bring about the greatest healing."

— Joshua Kai, The Quantum Prayer

Physical immunity is well known. The lesser-known but equally important one is emotional immunity. It can only be achieved when you understand the mind. Our mind is a faculty of consciousness and thoughts. Thoughts generate feelings and emotions. Negative and depressing thoughts generate negative emotions and feelings, thus impacting our emotional immunity and emotional health.

Emotional health is the ability to control negative emotions in a positive way such that we respond and not react. High energy emotions release positive neurotransmitters that send positive signals to every cell in the body which expedites healing. Similarly, low energy emotions have negative effects and cause diseases.

Our thoughts influence our physical health. Positive thoughts generate positive emotions thus helping us heal faster. Whereas, vibrations from thoughts and words of being unwell slow it down.

"Your thoughts are like a magnet, you attract what you think".

-Andrew Matthews

Once there was a strike of ambulance operators. Statistics reported by hospitals showed that emergencies had reduced drastically during the strike. Why? Because people had unconsciously started thinking that they would not get any ambulance service during the strike, so rather remain healthy.

Apart from medications, the family plays a huge role in the healing and curing of the patient. Not only our thoughts and words but also the collective vibrations of our family radiate through our entire body. We and our family need to consciously create healing and high energy thoughts.

Modern medical science gives importance to the role of the psyche in the process of healing cancer. This branch is known as psychiatric or clinical psycho-oncology.

In a recent study, 38% of cancer patients across India were found to have identifiable clinical anxiety or depressive disorder. A significant association between stressors and the progression of cancer has been observed for a long time. Studies have found increased stressful life events in the year before the diagnosis of breast cancer. In breast cancer, stressful events like bereavement or loss of a job were also associated with relapse. Stress can lead to immunosuppression. Surveys have found that 20-40% of patients show a significant level of distress.

With my research and experience I understood that if my psyche can cause the disease, it can also heal it. I realized that I would have to work on my psyche because the mind either heals or destroys the body. So, I started working on my emotional health to remove the blockages in the subtle energy. I focussed more on the various positive relaxation techniques most of which are spiritual but scientific. In this chapter, I will discuss two ways of increasing emotional immunity- first, affirmations and second, taking care of our karma to beget blessings and energy for healing.

A: Affirmation

Affirmations are a powerful reminder of the unlimited potential that resides within us. Most successful people in the society, like Mohammad Ali or Jim Carrey, the Hollywood superstar, used the "affirmation" technique to achieve sky rocking successes.

Whether you realise it or not, you are constantly having an internal dialogue in your head. Surprisingly, most of those thoughts are negative and wasteful. Patients with major illnesses, especially, have a negative image of the future. Negative self-talk releases negative hormones that impact the future of the disease. The vicious circle never breaks. Positive affirmations rewire your brain.

What exactly is an affirmation?

The affirmation can be defined as a consciously focused daily repetition of positive thoughts and words of health, happiness and relationships. They have a dramatic effect on our bodies if combined with visualisation and feeling. This technique is very useful in healing any disease. The mind can bring about physical changes in the body like reducing extra fat, increasing muscular strength and so on. Dr. Keith Clark conducted a study of 20 women in 1989 in which they used visualization techniques to have the desired figure. Without any suggestions on diet and exercise, the technique brought about a significant reduction in various parts of their bodies.

Pre-requisites for affirmations

Affirmations should be practised at least 3 to 4 times daily. Preferably, at the same time and the same place.

- It should not be a mindless repetition of phrases without any feeling.
- Affirmation should be in the present tense. For example, I am happy and healthy, I have abundant energy.
- It is more effective if practised in the morning and night before going to bed.

My Affirmations

The moment I open my eyes in the morning, I wish good morning to God. I repeat the affirmations in the present tense in my mind. I meditate visualizing myself as a healthy person. I also repeat the affirmations in bed right before falling asleep. My affirmations look something like this-

- I am healthy and healed
- God's purity is purifying diseased cells in my body
- My diseased cells are getting replaced with healthy cells
- My immunity power is increasing

My process

I combine my affirmation ritual with visualisations.

Putting my hands out with palms facing up, I visualize and feel powerful healing rays emerging from the Supreme healer (who is like micro-conscient light) falling on my palms. I then move my hands above my body, often making sweeping hand motions. These rays are healing my body. I then repeat the affirmations with the same feeling. This process doesn't take more than 5 minutes.

After my morning meditation, I drink one glass of warm water with raw turmeric. I then put positive affirmations in the water. While drinking I visualise the same feelings. While taking a bath and even when in the loo I visualise that all my diseased cells have washed away.

A scientific study of thoughts and words on water and food

A scientist from Japan, Masaru Emoto, proved that the molecular structure of water is changed by the presence of human conscious-ness nearby. This study has been backed by "exhaustive research". Masaru Emoto carried out very interesting experiments with water at the critical point for freezing. He claims that words expressing emotions affect the water crystals formed in the process. Emoto reports that words with positive emotional content produce beautiful crystals and those with negative emotional content generate ugly ones. Music and pictures are also reported to have similar effects. **Fig 4.1** (Courtesy: Internet)

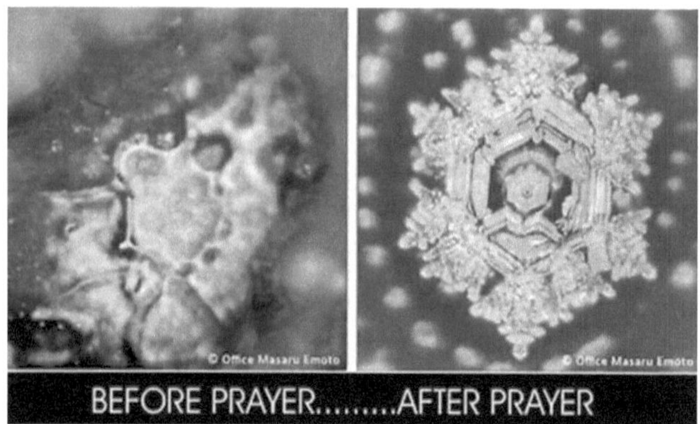

(Fig 4.1)

The miraculous subconscious mind

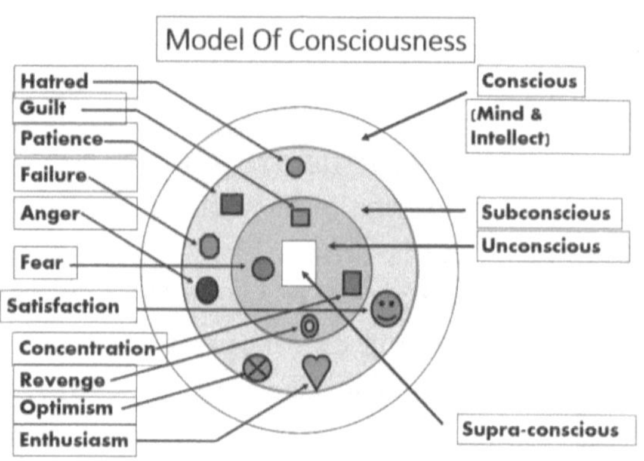

(Fig 4.2)

Our mind has two parts. The logically conscious mind (mind and intellect) makes up 20% of the mind. The remaining 80% is the subconscious (*sanskars*). **(Fig 4.2)** The subconscious mind is like an uneducated servant. It has no logic. It should be clearly understood that the mind is different from the 'brain'. The brain is the hardware and is made up of 100 billion neurons. There is the higher brain: the 2 cerebral hemispheres and the lower brain: the midbrain, pons, and medulla. The mind is the software and consists of thoughts, emotions, attitudes and memories.

The subconscious mind stores your beliefs, your previous experiences and your memories. All positivity and negativity are stored in the subconscious mind. If you believe that you are sick and weak you will feel the sickness. If your subconscious mind believes that you are healthy, you will heal because the body cells then start working in healing mode.

The moment the word cancer enters the mind, the subconscious mind due to the previous programming starts believing that this life has been cancelled. However, repeating positive words with faith makes the subconscious mind believe that you are healthy. The words enter and reprogram the subconscious mind and it starts working like a miracle.

Martin Brofman, the author of several books on healing, was diagnosed with terminal cancer of the spinal cord in 1975. He cured himself by using his consciousness to reprogram his mind. While eating he would imagine that the food is helping in healing cancer. He had positive fifteen-minute self-talks three times a day. By focusing his mind sharply on healing by visualisation and positive affirmations he cured himself completely.

B: Blessings and the law of karma

Blessings should be considered 'second medicine' in healing any disease. I truly felt that blessings contributed the most to my healing. It is rightly said - "*When medicines don't work blessings do.*"

Blessings are the return of the positive energy that you once gave to society and to nature. Blessing the world comes easily to me. Bless every person, situation and nature. Blessings or positive energy can also be received during your meditation practice from the Supreme healer, God.

My experience with blessings

I used to see many gynae-cancer patients when I started my gynaecological practice, mostly uterine cancer of the cervix (lower part of the uterus) and endometrium in the advanced stages. Because I could not do much for them, I always had compassion and would refer them for radiotherapy in higher centres. I never took any fees for their examination. Right after my post-graduation, I pledged to never charge any cancer patient. I believe that turned into a boon for me. This positive action balanced my negative karmic account that had caused cancer. I did not need to spend any finances on my treatment. I practically experienced the 'law of karma' in my own life.

My chemotherapy and radiation therapist, Prof. Dr. Shyamji Rawat, follows the same Brahma Kumaris organization that I do. He would say, "I am here for you, you don't need to bring anyone for your care." Even my surgery was performed by surgeons who follow the same spiritual teachings. I felt that God was treating and caring for me through his angels. The moment I realised that blessings are a boon in life, I focussed more and more on this aspect. I decided that for the rest of my life I would spend more time and energy on the welfare of society. This spiritual version taught at the Brahma Kumaris motivated me the most-

> *"If you use your body in service of humanity your body will be healthy, if you wish good luck for everyone your mind will be healthy, if you use your money for charity you will never have to ask for money, you will have in abundance not only in this birth but for many births. Those who spend time in spiritual service, their future will never be wasted solving trivial things."*

God blesses us in many ways. He wants to make us ever more powerful. However, at times, especially when cancer strikes, we doubt His intentions and may ask, "God! Why me?" Had we ever considered asking the same question when we had health, family and achievements? Then why now? He can only bestow blessings upon us, He can only protect us **(Fig 4.3)**.

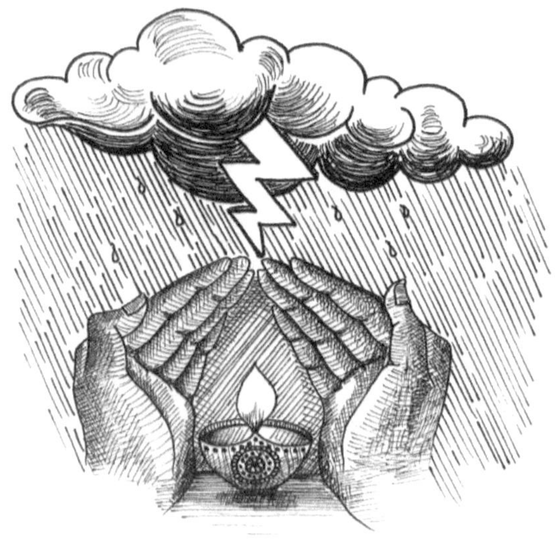

(Fig 4.3)

We should experience His blessings. The sufferings are a boon in disguise. It is rightly said, "God creates our fortune but it is us humans who spoil it."

Arthur Ashe was an American professional tennis player who has won three Grand Slam singles titles. He was a mixed-race African-American and had millions of fans all over the world. He was mistakenly given AIDS-infected blood during heart surgery in 1983. During the illness, he received a lot of letters from his fans, one of which asked:

"Why did God have to select you for such a bad disease?"

He was a thorough gentleman, to this Arthur replied -

50 million children started playing tennis, 5 million learnt to play tennis, 500,000 learnt professional tennis, 50 thousand came to the circuit, 5 thousand reached Grand Slam, 50 reached Wimbledon, 4 reached the semi-finals, 2 reached the finals and while holding the trophy in my hand, I never asked God: "Why me?" So now that I'm in pain how can I ask God: "Why me?"

Happiness ... keeps you sweet!

Trials ... keep you strong!

Sorrows ... keeps you human!

Failure ... keeps you humble!

Success ... keeps you glowing!

But only, Faith ... keeps you going!

Sometimes you are not satisfied with your life, while many people in this world are dreaming of living your life.

A child on a farm sees a plane fly up above and dreams of flying, while the pilot on that plane sees the farmhouse and dreams of returning home.

That's life!

Enjoy yours! If wealth were the secret to happiness, then the rich should be dancing on the streets. But only poor kids do!

If power ensured security, then VIPs would have walked unguarded. But those who live simply, sleep more soundly.

If beauty and fame bring ideal relationships, celebrities would have had the best marriages!

Live simply, be happy! Walk humbly and love genuinely!

The Law Of Karma

"As you sow, so shall you reap."

The law of Karma or Karma Philosophy is the answer to "why me?" No one can escape the result of his karma. Past bad karma or negative energy may return in the form of sickness, financial or relationship problems. You cannot control the past but the present is in your hands. You can accumulate for the future with present-day good actions. After curing my illness I decided to put all OPD (outpatient department) charges in the charity box. I could see for myself how wonderfully that worked. I was inspired by a lady outpatient who I had examined sometime back. She said, "Ma'am whenever I get a fever or any medical problem, I put money in the charity box and tell God, you are my surgeon, you treat me. Really, ma'am, I feel relieved." At the time I could not believe it, but now I understand how the subtle energy returns to me and makes me healthy, wealthy and happy. The law of energy can only be clearly understood when you realise who you are.

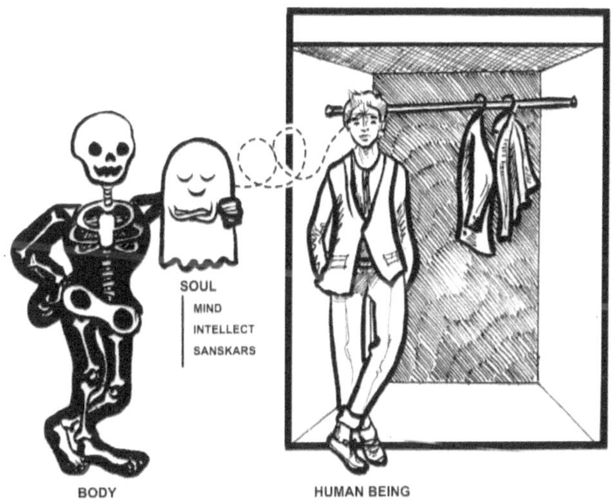

(Fig 4.4)

"You are a spiritual being having a human experience."

Human-being is derived from two Latin words, 'Humus' and 'Being'; humus means 'body' and being means 'psyche' or 'consciousness' or soul. As souls are on an unlimited journey and will take the next birth or body according to the karma we perform in the present life. There is no end to life. The body is like a costume. You change this costume again and again. The law of karma is inviolable. If not in this birth, then in the next, but the soul must and will receive the result or fruit of its karma (**Fig-4.4 and Fig 4.5**). Depending on the bad or good karma or action, one will suffer or enjoy, either in this or the next life. Now you should do the right karma that may create miracles in your life. In this birth when you leave your body you will be happy and content that you've done something noble for society. Past birth regression therapy, near-death experiences, out-of-body experiences and past birth memories cases support the existence of the soul. Past birth regression therapy helps in curing many diseases.

What is wrong *Karma*? You must acquire the right knowledge of what is good and what is bad action. Wrong karma is when someone acts, thinks or speaks under the influence of body consciousness (i.e. the five vices). Hence, everyone must act with a sense of consciousness.

What is Right karma? On the other hand, right karma is when a person has a balanced judgment, stability of mind, peace of the spirit and acts with the feeling of love, justice, sympathy, humility and performs his actions in a soul-conscious stage. Every human being is made up of two components viz. body and the soul. The real SELF is spirit. The soul is eternal and immortal, whereas, the body is mortal. When we think, speak and act with the consciousness of being a soul and consider this body merely an instrument, our acts are deemed good because such acts promote harmony, peace, unity and happy feelings. This can be practised by karma-yoga.

What is Karma Yoga?

Karma Yoga is to fulfil all your responsibilities without getting attached to them. Attachment causes anxiety. Any action performed with a pure intention benefits the self, then others and then spreads happiness to the world. Such action then certainly becomes a righteous deed. To perform righteous deeds or karma-yoga-

- Become trusty, surrender everything and every relation to God.
- Surrender the result of every action to God.

- Perform every action in a soul-conscious stage.
- Remember God while doing every karma.
- Give happiness to others.
- Perform karma for the benefit of others.
- Pray for the successes of others and enjoy others' successes.
- Offer food to God. Give peaceful and loving vibrations to food and water while cooking and eating.

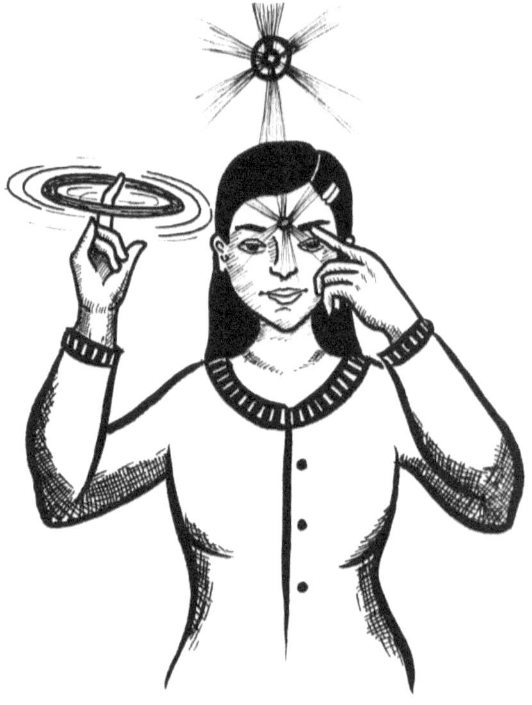

(Fig 4.5)

How I practice Karma Yoga

I never once asked the question, "Why me?" I treated the disease as an opportunity to settle my past karmic account. Throughout the treatment, I never had any stress or fear of the future or consequences. This was only possible because of the constant practice and awareness of the soul. I had always felt God's protective aura around me while performing any karma.

I shied away from anything trivial and took up more creative things. Deep down, in my subconscious, I knew that only the best would happen, no more, no less.

"You have to do the right thing. It may not be in your power, may not be in your time, that there'll be any fruit. But that doesn't mean you stop doing the right thing. You may never know what results come from your actions. But if you do nothing, there will be no result."

-M.K.Gandhi

Summary

- Daily positive affirmations with visualisation have a healing effect on any drastic disease.
- Blessings are the 'second medicine' for healing the mind and body in any illness.
- Understanding the law of karma is necessary for getting the answer to "why

me?" Good actions neutralize the past negative energy of bad actions and make you hopeful and happy.

Chapter 5

My Emotional DeTox

"The more the distance from negativity, the closer you are to happiness"

-Brahma Kumaris

Our atmosphere is increasingly becoming toxic, not only from the release of toxic gasses but also from the growing burden of negative vibrations. Poisoned feelings in human hearts have maligned and imbalanced the five elements of nature, of both the outer universe and our bodies. To restore the balance there is an urgent need to clean the blockages of the mind and body and get rid of toxic thoughts about yourself, others or the past. It is the call of time to internally detoxify and to put the outer (planet) and inner (body) nature in order. The theme of World Health day 2022 was "Our planet, Our Health". There is an urgent action needed to "keep humans and the planet healthy".

A. Forgiveness

"Forgiveness is no longer an option but a necessity for healing"

-Caroline Myss

An engineer with liver cancer once came to me for counselling and learning meditation. After the session, he asked, "Can negative feelings against someone be the cause of my cancer?"

My answer may not be obvious but conveys an important message, "Yes! Negative feelings like jealousy, hatred or animosity can all be the origin of cancer. All the systems of our bodies work as a unit. All cells of the bodywork in harmony, if we have jealousy for someone then these cells also feel jealous of each other and may cause neoplastic growth."

He then opened up about his inner feelings. He said in a distress, "I am the older of us two brothers. My parents gave all our parental property to my younger brother because he suffers from a cardiac problem. I haven't uttered a word about this to him, but inside I've been jealous of him ever since. I am a senior engineer and financially stable. Even though he has been in financial trouble I could not resist not feeling jealous. He has deceived me. I've not spoken to him since."

I explained to him, "You should forgive him because forgiveness is an act of self-service, more than anything else. The moment you forgive him, you will let go of the sad and acidic emotions that you have accumulated inside, thus releasing you of your damage. You can untangle yourself from the unhappy impressions stored in your memory and begin with a clean slate. Ask yourself, how long do you want to suffocate yourself for someone else's wrong behaviour? Should you continue the blame game or should you be healing yourself?"

I further said, "You should have mercy on him."

He asked why!

I introduced him to the spiritual law of Karma, "Your brother has financial problems but you are in such a highly respected position, probably because of your good karma. It is this understanding of the law of karma that ensures that every guilty person is punished, and the good ones rewarded. This universal law operates with impartiality. A feeling of mercy naturally emerges when you understand this law deeply. When you are wrong, you go to God for mercy and ask for the strength to face the fruit of your karma. He gives you strength, unconditional love and support to face it. (**Fig 5.1**) He expects you to follow the same path to forgive and support others. Repeat to yourself-

I am well-off, I am happy, I am content. Give him blessings, forgive him, talk to him and only then will you be happy! This will also help you heal."

I gave him the example of Brandon Bays, a motivational speaker. She is the world's leading authority on emotional healing and life transformation, author of 'The Inner Journey' and a lifestyle therapist for 18 years. She developed a football-sized cancerous pelvic tumour at the age of 39 years. She had undergone child abuse and domestic violence. But she healed herself by forgiving her parents and through emotional healing practices. The tumour got softened and she was tumour-free in six weeks. She also took colon therapy and a natural diet.

It has been studied that long-term resentment, disappointment and hopelessness cause cancer. Forgiveness is easy if you can forget the past and toxic feelings. It is easier said than done, practically, it takes time. I had similar feelings when I shifted to a new town. However, with daily spiritual and meditation practices, I could forgive the concerned person. I deeply practice this spiritual sentence in my life - "We do not have to take revenge, rather we have to change ourselves."

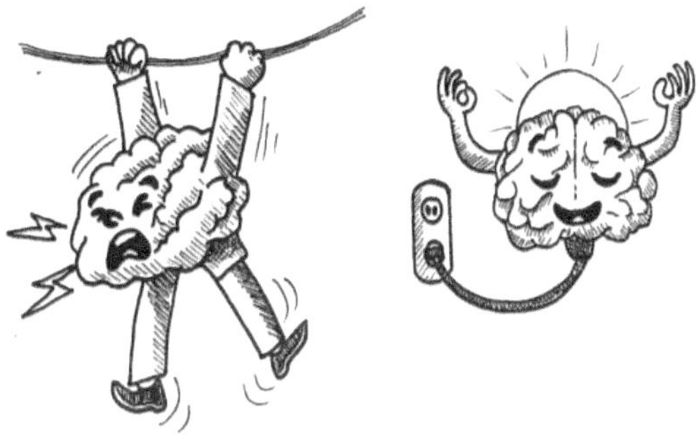

(Fig 5.1)

His inquisitive engineer brain continued to contemplate and he asked, "How can I do it when I see him again? Should I repeat the same thoughts in my mind?"

I asked him to practice meditation every day and in the last few minutes visualize and detoxify himself by saying with feeling–

I, the soul, am a child of God, I am the embodiment of love and peace.
I am a great soul. I have the strength of peace, love and joy.
The light of my soul is spreading everywhere.

Then, bring forth the person you have bitter feelings for. Imagine a star shining on their forehead and say–

My bitterness towards that soul is dissolving. With my heart, I forgive this soul.

I am feeling light. I am an angel.
I am spreading the rays of love and joy to the whole world.
I forgive him for his mistakes. My mind is clean.
I radiate love and respect to everyone.

How to forgive me for my mistakes?

Sometimes you have to forgive yourself. We all make mistakes knowingly or unknowingly. Here is a process I use to forgive myself- I apologize for my mistakes, if possible. I never postpone saying sorry. If I cannot reach out to seek forgiveness, I write a letter to the Supreme whom we call 'Baba' meaning Father and never feel the guilt.

A few years back a young lady came to me after a public program on meditation and said, "Ma'am I have been in depression for the last three years. I am a software engineer in Hyderabad. I am lucky to have a cooperative husband. Everything is great, but I have had some guilt since childhood. I feel very low and now I have developed depression."

I asked, "What happened in your childhood?".

She narrated in despair, "My parents were well-off, but my father was very arrogant. He would constantly quarrel with my mother. To avoid such disturbances, my mother would often send me to my grandfather's house to sleep.

One night I felt as if someone was inappropriately touching me. Much to my shock, that was my grandfather. I immediately informed my mother about the incident. My mom complained about this to my father. Instead of supporting us, he started abusing me and my mother. Since then I have been feeling guilty about telling my mother. I think because of this guilt I developed depression."

I counselled her with these words, "You were right about informing your mother or else the incidents would have kept happening. Now, because you have told me, your guilt will fade away. Telling someone is half the job done. Don't blame yourself, first love yourself and forgive everyone."

She was happier when she met me after a few days of learning meditation.

"There is no love without forgiveness, and there is no forgiveness without love."

- Bryant H. McGill

B. Gratitude

"An attitude of gratitude goes a long way when it comes to physical and emotional healing."

-Jill Bolte Taylor

Gratitude is to be grateful for everything you have in your life. It is a feeling of thankfulness towards the universe, every individual and the five elements of nature. It is the antidote to envy, hostility, worry and irritation. The moment you start thanking everyone, the 'law of attraction' starts working in your life. As a result, the universe starts taking care of you because 'positivity attracts positivity.' You will automatically get peace, happiness and love in your life. Therefore, this is one of the best methods to detoxify yourself.

We should express gratitude not only to people but also to things. Thus, you will create beautiful karma with objects, the house, car, mobile and everything that exists for us. This attitude of gratitude will finish your *sanskar* (habit) of complaining and criticizing.

Making gratitude a daily practice is like taking vitamins, the Vitamin-G tablet, says David Destine, professor in psychology at Northeastern University in Boston and the author of the book 'Emotional Success'. (**Fig 5.2**)

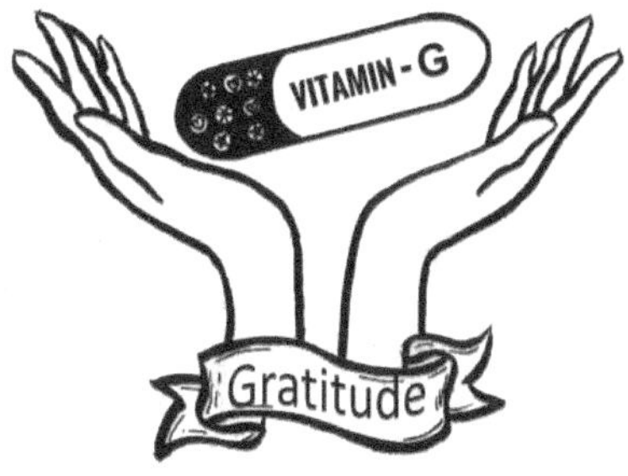

(Fig 5.2)

Robert Emmons, a professor in psychology at the University of California and the author of the book, "The Little Book of Gratitude", in one study, asked a group of volunteers to write down five things they are grateful for, once a week for ten weeks. The second group recorded either small hassles or neutral daily events. At the end of the study, the blessing counters reported feeling 25% happier and had fewer health complaints.

How do I practice?

Since childhood, I have felt deep compassion for the poor. I never asked God for anything when I visited temples even as a child. Instead, I would thank Him for what he had given me, then I would request Him to create a world where no one could be poor. Finally, in 1986, my happiness knew no bounds when I took a spiritual discourse from Brahma Kumaris. That is when I came to know that a beautiful world is about to come. There I learned the method of expressing gratitude toward everything. I used these learnings in my cancer healing process.

Every day after meditation and affirmation I practice gratitude towards–

My Body: "I thank you dear body, as you have helped me a lot in my life. I could study medical science through you! I even got this beautiful spiritual knowledge through you!"

My mind: "I thank you, my mind that I can focus on good things".

Wealth: "I thank you, wealth because you have maintained your balance enough to fulfil my basic needs."

Relatives: I thank my relatives without any judgement. This helps me progress in my life. I do this at a subtle level with real feelings every morning.

God: I thank God for He has given me everything in abundance. At times a positive outcome took time, but eventually, I could see that He gave me the best. This story beautifully expresses the feeling-

Once upon a time, there was a small kid who heard that God was distributing apples to humans in heaven. The kid was so happy to receive the news that he went to heaven with a lot of excitement to get the Apple from Him. However, there was a long queue. The kid joined the queue. When it was his turn, God gave the apple in his hands, but unfortunately, the Apple fell and got wasted in mud. The kid got disappointed and wondered, "What sin have I committed? I should suffer for it alone". He didn't want to return to earth with empty hands so he decided to stand in the queue for the second time.

This time the queue was even longer than the previous one. When his turn came, God put the apple in the kid's hand and spoke, "My dear child, the last time after giving you the apple I noticed that it was rotten and so I made it fall from your hands. I wanted to give you the best apple from my farm. At that time, the best on the farm was still growing and that is why I made you stand in the queue for a longer time. The apple that I just gave you is the best one grown on the farm to date. Enjoy it my child!"

Gratitude Practice

"I am a loving being. I thank God for what I have. I thank everyone whom I met and everything I used today. I thank the elements of nature for sustaining me today. I thank my body for being healthy today."

Purpose of life and Giving attitude

The purpose of human life is to find the answer to, "Why am I here?". In spiritual teachings, I learned that we are here to experience happiness by sharing, caring and cooperating with others, which means sharing what we have with everyone. **(Fig5.3)**

Giving attitude creates happiness in our lives. By replacing the energy of taking by giving good wishes through mind, sweetness through words and happiness through elevated deeds, anyone can notice a positive shift in a day, a week or a month with regular practice. After getting the disease I have been focussing more on giving. Now, the aim of my life is to give. I try to spread well wishes to everyone, I take care of my words and help everyone as much as possible. I felt that a giving attitude gave me immense happiness and detoxified me. This service keeps me so busy that I do not get any time for worry or tension.

"The happiest people in life are givers, not takers"

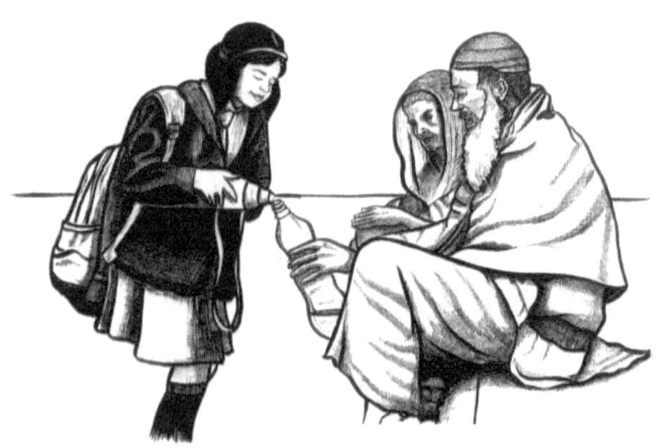

(Fig 5.3)

Once a king was donating to all his subjects. A beggar was standing in the queue to collect the donation. However, as soon as the beggar's chance would come he would go back to rejoin the queue.

Everyone was surprised that a beggar was doing this!

On asking he replied, "I noticed that the king gets happy each time he donates. I wanted to experience that too. Although I don't have anything physical to give, I do have a chance to get a donation. Every time I give that chance away to the next one in the queue I feel happy."

In his book "Why Good Things Happen to Good People", Stephen Post, a professor of preventive medicine at Stony Brook University, writes that giving to others has been shown to increase health benefits and longevity in people with chronic illnesses.

A 1999 study led by Doug Oman of the University of California, Berkeley, found that elderly people who volunteered for two or more organizations were 44 per cent less likely to die in five years than were non-volunteers, even if they had been practising exercise, maintaining general health, and following negative health control habits like smoking.

Stephanie Brown of the University of Michigan saw similar results in a 2003 study on elderly couples. She and her colleagues found that people who provided practical help to friends, relatives, or neighbours, or gave emotional support to their spouses, had a lower risk of dying in five years than those who did not. Interestingly, receiving help was not linked to reduced death risk.

Researchers suggest that one reason why giving may improve physical health and longevity is that it helps decrease stress, which is one of the causes of various health problems. In a 2006 study by Rachel Piferi of Johns Hopkins University and Kathleen Lawler of the University of Tennessee, it was found that people who provided social support to others had lower blood pressure than participants who did not, suggesting a direct physiological benefit to those who give of themselves.

"Life is a gift. Wake up every morning and realize that."

Summary

- Detoxification of toxic thoughts is necessary. Toxic thoughts cause blockage in the subtle aura and delay healing.
- Forgiveness is very easy and detoxifies you when you understand the law of karma

- Gratitude and giving attitude help in emotional and physical healing

Chapter 6

Are Genes My Destiny?

"In every human being, genomes tell the story of our evolution, written in the language of DNA. The narrative is unmistakable and ever-changing."

— Michael Corthell

"Ma'am, I've seen my father and three brothers suffering and dying of cancer. I am always scared, doctor. Do I have the same fate?" Every time she met me, she would ask me this question.

Indeed, such questions are worth considering. If genes are my destiny, do my parents have the potential to destine my disease? Can I control pre-programmed gene maps which are set at my birth? Do we have any control over the genes that they are expressed in, and do they stay dormant? If the family tree has cancer, can you turn off genes that have a negative effect on us?

Science now says that you have the power to modify your genes by altering your diet and adopting an active and stress-free life. With these positive life changes, you can have control of "gene expression" which can change the destiny of any disease. This is termed as "Epigenetics."

In February 2022, I lectured on "Healthy Lifestyle to Prevent Cancer" to celebrate World Cancer Day. The most common question asked that day was- "What precaution should I take if I have a family history of cancer?"

The prior aim of this chapter is to make you realize that the most common myth about cancer is that if you have a family history you are bound to get cancer. Your healthy lifestyle can modify the gene expression and you have the potential to switch off unhealthy genes.

Epigenetics

About 65-75% of people in a village in Sweden have cancer, with every sixth woman suffering from breast cancer. In a peculiar case, although the disease was prevalent in the family there was one senior member who did not have cancer. How come a single family member is exempt from cancer? Science could not ascertain if the gene was present in the family. Research, popularly known as the 'Human Genome Project', was conducted to identify the cause behind this anomaly. This study led to the discovery of epigenetics.

Genes and epigenetics

I will only touch upon the basics of genes and epigenetics. A basic understanding is necessary because science now says that the signals from epigenomes change the way genes are regulated.

The human body is composed of around a trillion cells. A cell has many parts, one of which is the nucleus. Within the nucleus, the human genome contains 3 billion base pairs which reside in 23 pairs of chromosomes that are a complete set of DNA. (**Fig-6.1**)The gene is the smallest segment of DNA. Gene is the basic functional and physical unit of heredity. Gene carries information that determines your trait. 25,000-35,000 genes make only 5% of the genome, the rest consists of switches, the epigenome - a network of chemical compounds surrounding the DNA that modify the genome without altering the DNA sequences. The epigenome plays a role in determining which genes are active in a particular cell. Imagine a 100 pages long book in which the first 95 pages are instructions (i.e. epigenome) on how to read the book.

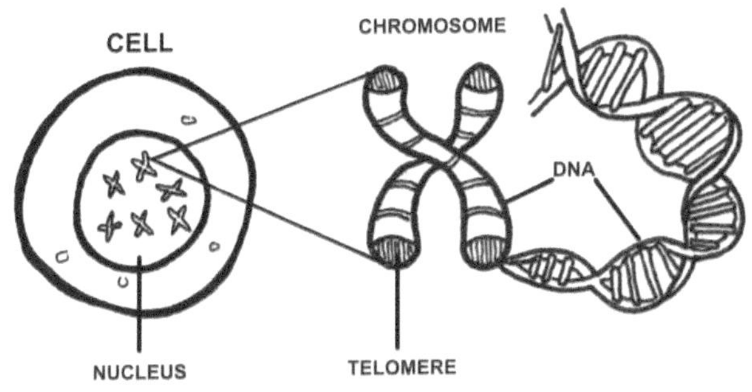

(Fig. 6.1)

Epigenetics is on top of genetics. Whether you will have cancer or not, depends on which gene is "turned on" and which gene is "turned off". This subject is called "epigenetics". Epigenetics doesn't change the genetic code, rather, it changes how it is read. Epigenetics can be defined in easy language as the external factors like diet, exercise, thoughts or meditation that change the expression of genes negatively or positively mainly during in-utero and childhood.

What affects the epigenome?

Biologists say that if the genome is the hardware, then the epigenome is the software. The Times magazine published an article in January 2010 on "Why your DNA isn't your destiny" exploring the findings from Dr. Lars Olov Bygren's research on epigenetics. He discovered that dietary and lifestyle conditions not only affected the genetic expression of each individual but also of their children and grandchildren. He concluded, "It is through epigenetic marks that environmental factors like diet, stress and prenatal nutrition can make an imprint on genes that are passed from one generation to the next."

Epigenetic changes to chromatin (a substance within a chromosome consisting of DNA and protein) may result from

- Development in utero,
- Childhood,
- Environmental chemicals,
- Drugs,
- Ageing,
- Diet, exercise,
- Thoughts and meditation.

These changes result in cancer and many autoimmune diseases.

The agouti mouse model depicts that a little change in diet during pregnancy can change the destiny of the offspring. Back in 2000, Randy Jirtle, a professor of radiation oncology at Duke University, and his postdoctoral student Robert Waterland proved this by scientific experiment. They started with pairs of fat yellow mice known to scientists as agouti mice because these mice carry a particular gene - the agouti gene which is prone to cancer and diabetes. (**Fig 6.2**) The aim was to see if they could change the agouti gene expression of these mice. They changed the mother's diet starting just before conception. Jirtle and Waterland fed a test group of mother mice a diet rich in methyl donors. Hypomethylation activates oncogene and hypermethylation initiates the silencing of cancer-suppressing genes. These molecules are found in many foods, including onions, garlic, beets, and in the food supplements often given to pregnant women. After being consumed by the mothers, the methyl donors worked their way into the developing embryos' chromosomes and onto the critical agouti gene. The mothers passed along the agouti gene to their children intact, but due to their methyl-rich pregnancy diet, they had added to the gene a chemical switch that weakened the gene's deleterious effects. "How something as subtle as a nutritional change in the pregnant mother rat could have such a dramatic impact on the gene expression of the baby," Jirtle says. "The results showed how important epigenetic changes could be."

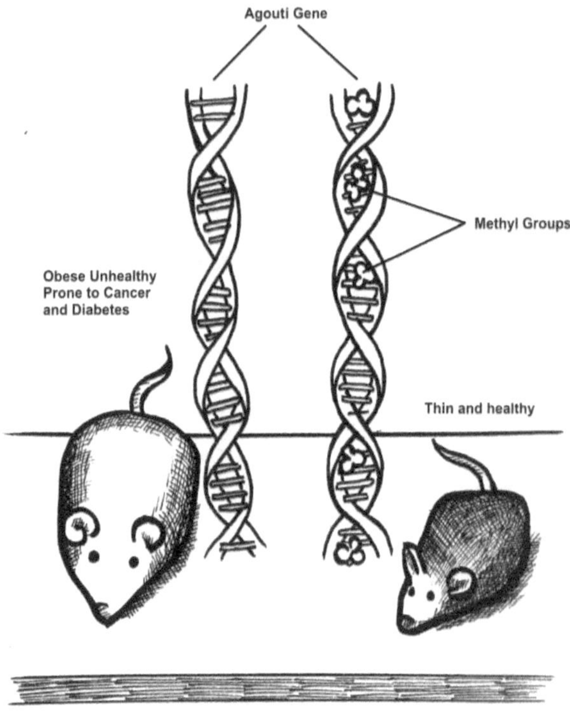

(Fig 6.2)

It is well known that the environment in a mother's womb, like stress and diet, can alter the development of a fetus. The epigenetic changes brought by one's diet, behaviour, or surroundings can work their way into the germline and echo far into the future. This means what you eat or smoke today could affect the health and behaviour of your great-grandchildren.

More and more researchers are finding that an extra bit of a vitamin, a brief exposure to a toxin and even an added dose of mothering can change the epigenome, and thereby alter the software of our genes in ways that affect an individual's body and brain for life. We commonly accept the notion that through our DNA we are destined to have particular body shapes, personalities, diseases and conventional wisdom, but many studies have now confirmed that epigenetic effects play a more important role than genes in developing any disease.

The Dutch Hunger Winter study- Food shortage and famines at the end of World War II impacted the children born during that period. It was found that those children had a twofold increase in mental disorders like schizophrenia, schizoid/ schizotypal personality disorder, as well as affective disorders in adulthood. These effects reflect specific biological mechanisms, possibly through the impact of the environment on the epigenome. Scientists have now discovered that the epigenome can change in response to the environment not only during early fetal development but also throughout an individual's lifetime.

"People used to think that once your epigenetic code was laid down in early development, that was it for life," says Moshe Szyf. "But life is changing all the time, and the epigenetic code that controls your DNA is turning out to be the mechanism through which we change along with it. Epigenetics can also be changed at any age by altering the environment, diet and thinking. It has been seen that separated identical twins reared in different environments constitute different individuals. Epigenetic patterns shift through life and those positive changes can even save lives.

This can be understood by the story of a living example published in the Irish Times- "The man who forgot to die".

Buettner interviewed Stomatis Moraitis, an Ikarian who emigrated to the US in 1943 and lived there until 1976 when he was diagnosed with lung cancer. He was given nine months to live. He returned to live his remaining months in Ikaria. Moraitis spent the first few months in bed, during that time he started taking healthy food and remained happy with his friends. Moraitis gradually recovered his strength, started to plant vegetables in his garden, enjoyed the sun and sea air, and reconnected with the <u>Greek Orthodox</u> faith of his youth.

Months passed by and Moraitis did not die; in fact, he grew stronger. He eased into the island routine. He rose from bed in the morning when he felt like it, worked in the garden and vineyard into the mid-afternoon, made lunch and then took a long nap.

The years passed and his health continued to improve. He never had chemotherapy or took any medicine. He simply moved home to Ikaria.

Buettner asked Moraitis how he got rid of his cancer. He replied, "It just went away. I went back to America about 25 years after moving here to see if the doctors could explain how it was cured." "Then what happened?" asked Buettner. "My doctors were all dead," said Moraitis. He passed away cancer free at the age of 102.

Epigenetics brings both good news and bad. Bad news first: there's evidence that lifestyle choices like smoking and eating too much can change the epigenetic marks on your DNA in ways that cause the genes for obesity to express themselves too strongly and the genes for longevity to express themselves too weakly. We all have genes that can cause or suppress cancer. However, we can activate switches (i.e. epigenomes that instruct genes) that activate tumour-suppressing genes. This can be achieved only with positive lifestyle changes.

A scientific study: Role of epigenetics in the development of cancer

Genes are the loaded gun for any disease and lifestyle is a trigger. Some genes can cause cancer, some genes can prevent cancer. Whether you will have cancer or not depends on which gene is turned on or off. Several research studies have proven the relationship between lifestyle and gene expression.

Dr. Dean Ornish and others from the Preventive Medicine Research Institute and the University of California (2011) found that meditation and a healthy lifestyle can even change genes related to cancer. They studied the effect of lifestyle changes in men with early-stage prostate cancer and found changes in over 500 genes. Many disease-promoting genes were turned off whereas protective, disease-preventing genes were turned on. (**Fig.6.3**)

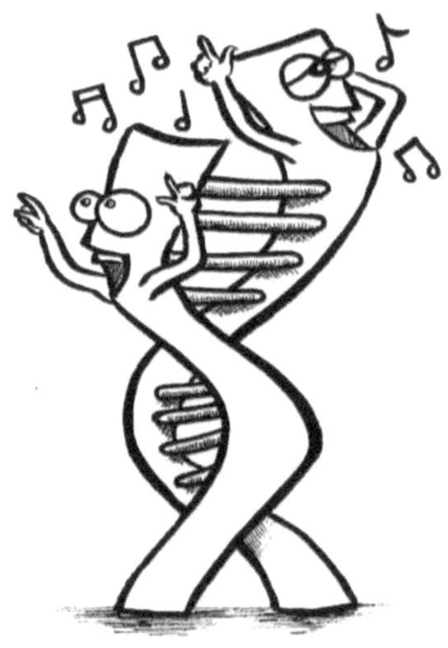

(Fig 6.3)

After practising meditation in prostate cancer RAS, a set of genes that can cause cancer was seen turned off. The E-selectin gene which promotes inflammation elevated in breast cancer was also found to be turned off. Another gene called SFRP that prevents tumour formation was seen turned on thereby reducing the risk of cancer.

Importance of Telomere length in Health

Telomeres are the protein caps at the end of chromosomes that determine how quickly cells age. Lifestyle changes the telomere length of chromosomes that are responsible for maintaining the health of DNA. You have the power to regulate telomere length. (**Fig6.4**)

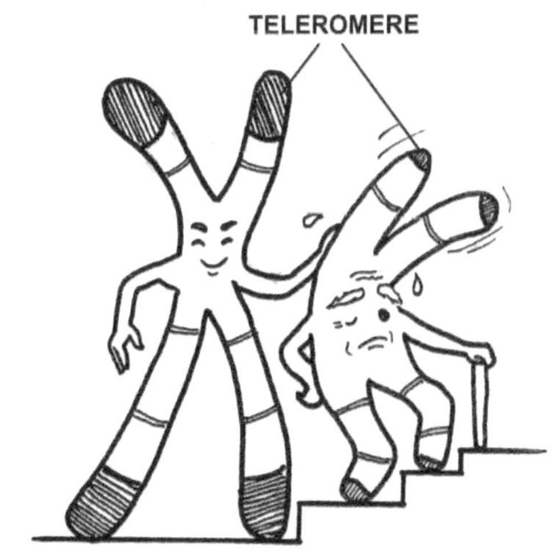

(Fig 6.4)

The study published in the journal *'Cancer',* *2014* was one of the first to suggest scientifically, that a mind-body connection does exist. The study included 88 breast cancer survivors who had completed at least three months of treatments. A subgroup met weekly for 12 weeks of follow-up mindfulness-based activities. The participants attended group discussions along with meditation and yoga sessions and committed to practising meditation and yoga at home for 45 minutes daily.

Following the study of this group, researchers found that the telomeres stayed the same length in cancer survivors who meditated or took part in support groups over the three months. On the other hand, the telomeres of a control group (the other subgroup) of cancer survivors who didn't participate in these groups, were shortened during the three-month study. Shortened telomeres are associated with several disease states, as well as cell ageing, while longer telomeres are thought to be protective against disease.

Telomere length predicts our lifespan or ageing and susceptibility to diseases. (**Fig 6.4**) Telomerase enzymes increase telomere length. Good nutrition, exercise, happiness, gratitude, positive thinking, self-love, and having a purpose in life increase telomere enzymes, thus increasing telomere length.

"Epigenetics reveals that we are not 'victims' of our genes but are in fact 'masters' of our genes."

- Bruce Lipton-PhD

Summary

- Genes are not my destiny. We have control over genes by adopting a healthy lifestyle i.e. epigenetics.
- Whether we will have cancer or not, depends on which gene is "turned on" and which gene is "turned off".
- Telomere length can be changed by a healthy lifestyle.
- Epigenetic changes are passed to generations **even** to grandchildren.

References

Obesity, Epigenetics, and Gene Regulation

By: Jill U. Adams, PhD (*Freelance Science Writer*) © 2008 Nature Education

Citation: Adams, J. (2008) Obesity, epigenetics, and gene regulation. *Nature Education* 1(1):128

Chapter 7

What Exactly Heals?

Soul or Body - Mind or Brain

"You are the creator of your world and the power of creation is in your thoughts."

-Brahma Kumaris

We have learned the importance of physical and emotional immunity so far. However, spiritual energy is equally crucial. Modern science defines health as the harmonious inflow of physical, emotional and spiritual energy. True healing starts from the spirit. Diseases occur when there is a blockage in spiritual energy reaching the cells of the body. Your spiritual energy is what forms your aura. It can be seen in Kirlian photography, a process that reveals visible "auras" around the objects photographed.

Doctors cannot say that you are cured of cancer, but if you remain in complete remission for at least 5 years chances of survival are more. To keep it at bay and eventually cure it for good, you have to go much deeper than just the physical and emotional realms and empower your inner selves' metaphysical energy.

Personally, whenever I am faced with a problem, I introspect, connect with my inner self and the Supreme, and voila I get the solution. This spiritual knowledge made me realize that the cause of my illness is at a metaphysical level. And so I started using this knowledge in my healing.

Everything in the universe is a system of energy. The human consciousness field has the soul as the highest and rarest form of energy, and the body is the densest. The mind which creates thoughts and emotions is also a part of metaphysical energy. i.e. the soul; the brain is only hardware. The soul creates reality in the physical dimension through the mind. The body is not the primary, which unfortunately in today's age has "somehow overpowered the mind and the soul". (**Fig 7.1**)

Mind over matter

What heals, Body or Mind?

True story- In 1957 a new medicine was experimented for the treatment of cancer. A patient with a big tumour in the neck read this report somewhere and asked his doctor, "Doctor, could you treat me with that injection,

Krebiozen, I might get cured?" The doctor agreed and a couple of doses of the injection were given to the patient. Soon the whole tumour melted like ice and he was cured for almost 6 months. The recovery was very dramatic. Six months later, he came across another report in the newspaper that the experiments carried out on the drug may not be effective after all because Krebiozen was not a good drug. Upon reading this, the patient magically developed the same tumour. He returned to the doctor and the doctor said, "We've found that the previous dose was not pure, let's give a second shot!" After the second trial, the patient again recovered until ultimately the final announcement came in the 'American Journal of Oncology' stating that Krebiozen was a useless drug and did not cure cancer. Soon after he succumbed.

This is a very famous example that has been quoted in many books on 'mind, body and medicine'. What does this imply? Who or what exactly was responsible for his momentary recovery? Indeed! His mind. It is the mind that can heal or even kill a person.

What is mind?
Are mind and body synonymous?

Mind	Brain
Software	Hardware
Non physical, abstract	Physical
T: Thoughts	100 billion neurons
E: Emotions	Higher brain: 2 cerebral hemispheres
A: Attitude	Lower brain: mid brain, pons, medulla
M: Memories	

(Fig 7.1)

Soul conscious lifestyle to heal the body

Our present healthcare system focuses only on treating physical diseases. Almost all research is focused on the processes in the physical body. But, are we just bodies, or are we something beyond the physical? We are **'Human Beings'**. It was only around 70-80 years back that dichotomy in the states of being of the 'Human Being' was emphasized. 'Human Being' is derived from two Latin words, 'Humus' and 'Being'; humus meaning 'body' and being meaning 'psyche' or 'consciousness'. This depicts the multi-dimensionality of a 'human being'. Care of the 'being' part is known as spiritual health. Spiritual Health refers to the part of an individual that reaches out and strives for meaning and purpose in life.

The first part of spirituality is to understand yourself and explore the purpose of life. Spirituality and religion are not synonymous. Religion stands for a group of people with a common belief system associated with rituals. Spirituality is not blind faith, it is a broader concept that aims to seek a meaningful connection with something bigger than yourself. It has the answers to deeper questions like, "Why did this happen to me?", "Am I going to die, is my future secure?", "Did God punish me?", "How can I be happy?".

A soul-conscious lifestyle takes charge of your mind and emotions by understanding the being and the soul. The soul is the metaphysical energy that controls the body. At the molecular and genetic level, 98% of the human body is replaced each year; what is continuous is the 'consciousness'. This consciousness recreates the body and the brain including the DNA. Past birth regression therapy and cases of near-death experiences confirm the existence of metaphysical energy.

Anatomy of soul

Human beings are made up of the soul and the body. The soul is like a seed of metaphysical energy and is located at the centre of the forehead, seated on the hypothalamus.

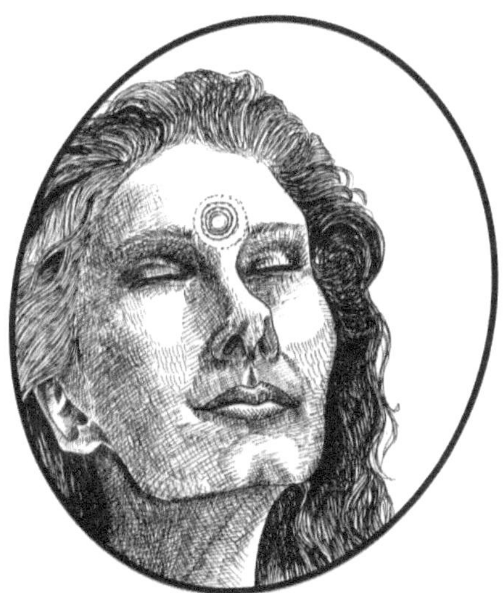

Physiology of soul

- The peaceful and serene soul has three faculties that are the subtle expressions of consciousness:
- The mind that creates thoughts, emotions and desires.
- The intellect that has the power to discern.
- The *sanskars* constitute our memories, impressions and habits.

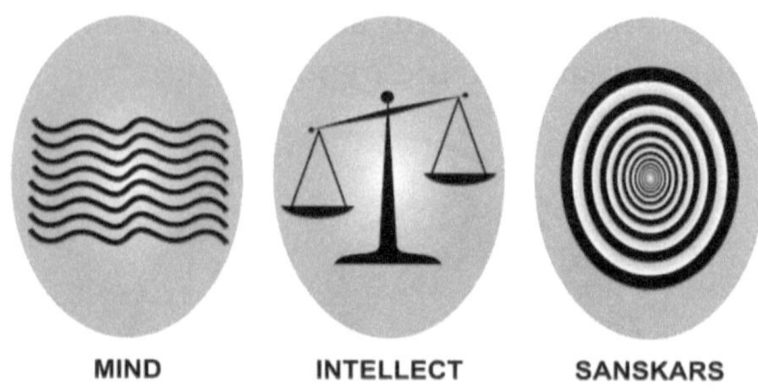

(Fig 7.2)

The soul has seven innate qualities, namely, knowledge, peace, love, purity, happiness, power and bliss (spiritual energy). The metaphysical energy acts through the mind, thoughts, judgements, feelings and emotions. and integrates with the biological energy of the body through the nervous and endocrine system, thereby, nourishing every cell of the body. Each cell of the body needs all the seven qualities of the soul, but every system of the body needs a different one the most. (**Table7.1**) A soul-conscious lifestyle enhances these qualities by creating positive thoughts, emotions, attitudes and memories that release positive chemicals in the body.

Table7.1

Physical energy	Metaphysical energy
Human, the body which is corporeal	Being, the soul which is incorporeal
Soil	Soul
Inert, physical	Conscious, metaphysical
Destructible	Imperishable
Visible	Invisible
Mine	I
Physical organ system	Innate qualities of soul Necessary for the health of physical body
5 sense organs and immune system	Purity
Respiratory and cardiovascular systems	Peace and love
Digestive system	Happiness
Central nervous system	Knowledge
Endocrine system, Genital system	Bliss
Musculoskeletal system	Power

Power of faith in the Higher-Self in Healing-

The second part of spirituality is to have faith in the Supreme. A connection with Him is necessary to enhance healing. Since the universe is immensely interconnected, the feeling of separateness (i.e. separateness of human beings from God, individuals from families, families from society) is a source of stress. We will have to understand Him to develop a relationship with Him and uproot this feeling of separateness.

What is His name? What are His qualities and form? God, or the Supreme, is a pure spirit and incorporeal, that is, He does not have any human or animal form. He is like a radiant invisible star of blissful light. He is a separate distinct being, who remains above and beyond, and is eternally free from any bondage to the material world. He is the ocean of knowledge, peace, purity, love, happiness, bliss and power. He is a father, a teacher, a guru and a true friend. With Him, you can experience any relationship you want.

During the treatment, I saw God as a 'Supreme Surgeon'. This connection made me strong and stress-free. The Supreme is a powerhouse. You will heal faster if you make a connection and pull His subtle energy for healing.

"I am a God-lover. I accept that God is one and a microcoscient light, but He is the almighty. I have full faith in Him. I have surrendered everything to Him."

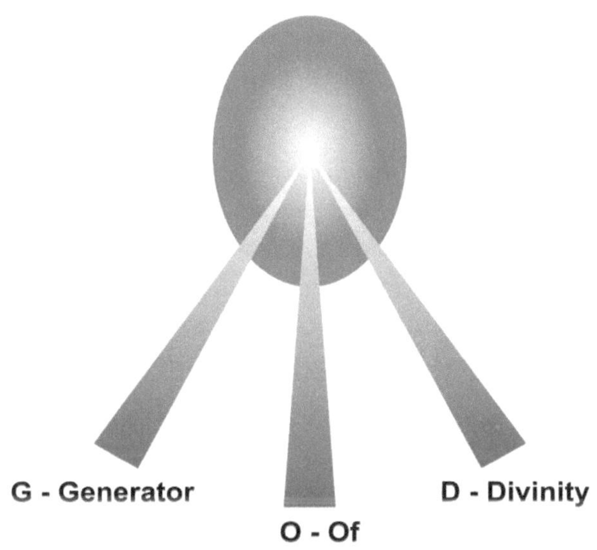

(Fig 7.3)

This feeling makes me fearless. No worries creep in because I have surrendered myself to God. I know that He had sent me many beautiful angels for my care in the form of divine surgeons, radiologists, and my divine family members. If you are connected with God, even your doctor shall be touched with the right thought at the right time to make the right decisions. Although spirituality is important for healing, you should not have blind faith. Treatment is of utmost necessity. I have seen many deceased patients who had wasted time consulting various doctors or refused treatment. They either have no faith in doctors or have blind faith in God. You can understand this more easily by relating this story-

Once there was a flood in a village and all the houses were submerged. Most people got away in rescue boats, some drowned. There was a man who managed to get to the top of the roof. He had an unwavering faith that God would save him from dying. He was praying to God for help.

Soon, a man in a rowboat came by and hollered, "Jump in man, I can save you."

The stranded man shouted back, "No, it's okay! I'm praying to God and he is going to save me."

So the rowboat went on.

A few moments later a motorboat came by. The fellow in the motorboat shouted, "Jump in man, I can save you."

To this, the stranded man said, "No thanks! I'm praying to God and he is going to save me. I have faith."

The motorboat went on.

Then a helicopter came by and the pilot called out, "Grab this rope and I will lift you to safety."

To this, the stranded man again replied, "No thanks! I'm praying to God and he is going to save me. I have faith."

So the helicopter reluctantly flew away.

Soon the water rose above the rooftop and the man drowned. He went to Heaven and finally got his chance to discuss this whole situation with God, at which point he exclaimed, "I had full faith in you but you did not save me after all, you let me drown. I don't understand why!"

To this God answered, "I sent you a rowboat, a motorboat and a helicopter, what more did you expect?"

Spirituality attenuates the fear of death. Many scientific studies prove that those who believe in God have less stress, feel more secure and have faster healing. Healing further reduces anxiety, fear and stress. Knowledge of immortality of the soul and connection with God reduces the fear of death. Fear of death is the first thought upon diagnosis of cancer. This fear releases toxins that eventually lead to recurrence or even death. Spirituality helps to cope with stress and makes the person fearless.

Once an epidemic hit a village. Soon villagers started dying. On seeing this the village saint asked her, "Why have you come?"

The epidemic roared, "I have come to take 100 of your people".

When it was time for the epidemic to return, the saint inquired, "How many people are you taking?"

She audaciously replied, "I am taking 10,000 people!"

Hearing that the saint accused her of lying, "You had said that you will take only 100 people away! Why did you not keep your promise?"

The pandemic laughed and said, "I had indeed come to take only 100 people, but the rest 9,900 perished due to fear."

This comes true in many diseases. During the second wave of covid in India, when the death rate was high, many patients died in hospitals due to fear just because the person next to them had succumbed.

On 6th February 2022, we organized a program for cancer survivors in the Brahma Kumaris organization. Around 60 patients took part in this program. They had all survived and their durations of cancer survival varied from 2 to 8 years. We asked them to fill out the following questionnaire-

How satisfied are you in life?

Do you believe in soul and karmic accounts?

- How much do you believe in God?
- Who do you think has treated you?
- What do you think is the reason you recovered?
    - Karma
    - Luck
    - Something else ________
- How interested are you in spiritual knowledge after recovery?
- Do you feel any stress post-recovery?

80% were satisfied. 92% per cent of those who believed in God also believed in soul and Karma. 70% believed that God treated the disease, whereas, 30% said the doctor. 20% felt bad luck got them cancer. Those who believed and had faith in God experienced lesser stress.

After the session I asked them, "How many of you are willing to serve the society?" Most of them raised their hands, but weren't sure how. It was evident that most of them had realised that after getting cancer life is more precious, and now they want to utilise their lives for the service of humanity. Exactly this is spirituality and the purpose of life - to serve society. There are many ways by which spiritual energy can be increased:

- Selfless service
- Prayer
- Belief in the Higher self
- Self-reflection
- Guided visualisation
- Yoga and meditation

"May you become full of the treasure of happiness and by keeping the awareness of having all attainments, kick away sadness."

-Brahma Kumaris

Summary

- Your mind has a tremendous power to heal your body.
- A soul-conscious lifestyle is a healthy lifestyle.
- An incurable disease means a disease that heals when you go deep inside and heal it from within.
- God is the ultimate power bank. Connect and draw from him to secure your future and live healthily and happily ever after.

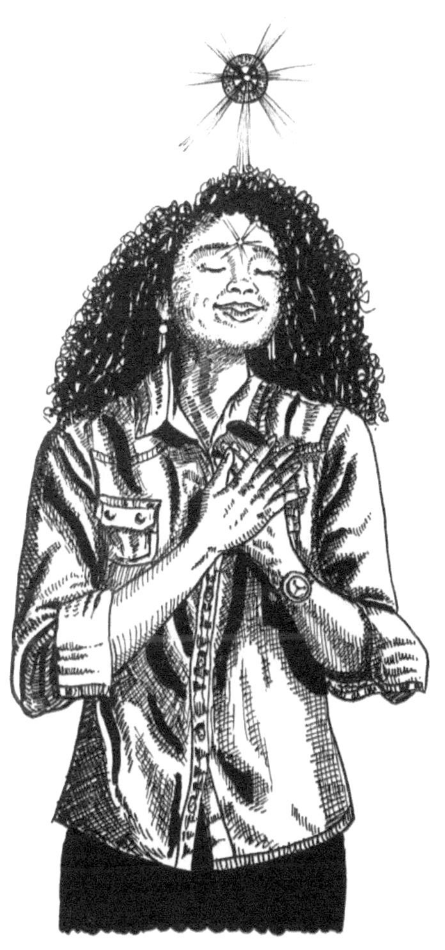

Chapter 8

Healing Meditation

"Who looks outside, dreams, who looks inside awakens."

- Carl Jung

One of my friends who is a senior gynaecologist also practices meditation. In one of the programs for cancer prevention, she shared a wonderful story of a 34-year-old lady, a known patient, depicting the healing effects of meditation. One day this patient came to see her and complained, "My *naani* and my mothers' eldest sister died due to breast cancer a few years back. My elder sister also had breast cancer, although she was operated for it, she ultimately died a few months back. Now, I'm the youngest in the family and very much disturbed as I can feel a nodule in my left breast."

Upon palpation, the gynaecologist found a 1cm firm lump present on the left side of the patient's breast and advised FNAC (biopsy) that showed positive for malignant cells. She advised an operation but the patient refused. So my doctor friend recommended, "Since you are going back to Bombay, try and find the Brahma Kumaris centre near your home, go and meet the Brahma Kumari sister and tell her all about your disease. Ask her to give you the seven-day course followed by sessions on healing meditation. Learn and practice meditation regularly with full faith in the Supreme and His healing energy." She did it.

"After 6 months when she visited me again, she had no lump. What a miraculous change!", the doctor said. The patient said with a sigh of relief, "Doctor, even though I was not feeling a lump, I wanted to get it checked by you properly." Follow-up mammography was done and no lump was present. The patient was very happy. This is a great example of the healing powers of meditation.

Another example is me. I practised this healing Rajyoga meditation to heal my body during the treatment and I am still continuing the meditation practice. Another patient, Usha Bai, who used to practice meditation was diagnosed with oesophagal cancer in the 3rd stage. In spite of the radiation, it recurred after 3 years, but she continued her meditation practice and now it has been 8 years, as of 2022, of wellness.

What is Meditation?

Meditation has come from the word *'medri'* which means 'to heal'. Meditation is a process of getting to know myself completely, both who I am 'inside' and how I react to what is 'outside'. You learn how to distinguish between the different thought patterns and how to select those patterns that are positively useful and help you achieve your goal.

Through meditation, I discovered a different me, from the stressed or troubled person who I thought I used to be. It helped me realise that my true nature is very positive.

Purpose of Meditation- I have been practising meditation for a long time, even before the disease. My aim was not the healing, but unknowingly it proved to be a boon at the time of my illness (**Fig8.1**). Meditation serves many purposes - few people meditate for better mental health, few for increasing concentration and some meditate to become calm and peaceful. Whatever the reason, the underlying purpose is spiritual. Patients who have been diagnosed with advanced cancers have their minds full of worry and stress. Meditation techniques help manage the stress of the illness by reducing the side-effects of the medical treatment and by giving a sense of being in control of the illness. All of this costs nothing. Meditation is one of man's most ancient activities. It is most probably the oldest known technique for self-healing.

ADD MEDITATION TO YOUR MEDICATION.

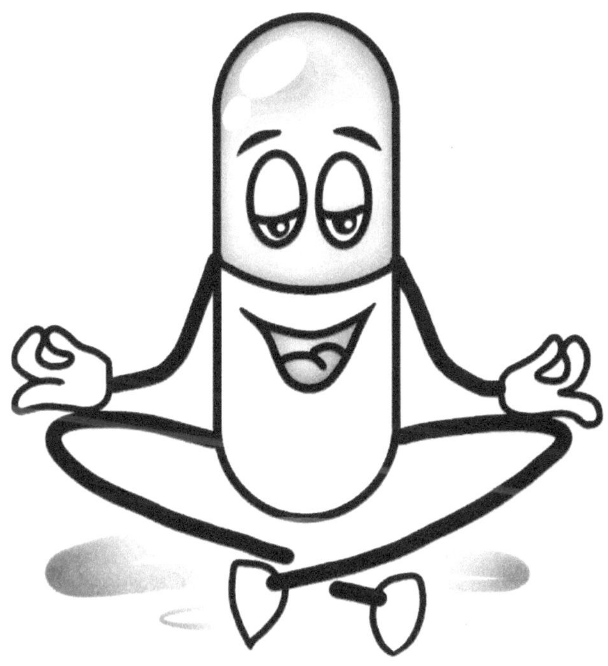

(Fig 8.1)

How meditation helps cancer patients

Stress Response and Yoga Response

	Stress Response	Yoga Response
Heart Rate	↑	↓
Blood Pressure	↑	↓
Respiration	↑	↓
Metabolism	↑	↓
Bad Cholesterol	↑	↓
Good Cholesterol	↓	↑
Blood Vessel Size	↓	↑
Skin Resistance	↓	↑
Brain Alpha Waves	↓	↑

References

- Patel Giresh- Effect of Rajyog Meditation on Vital Parameters, book Meditation as Medicine Mount Abu 1984

(Table 8.1)

Meditation reduces emotional and psychological stress (Table 8.1)-

Helps cure anxiety and chronic stress by decreasing metabolic rate and lowering the heart rate, thus indicating a state of deep rest and regeneration. Meditation reduces stress by decreasing stress hormones. It restores the functions of serotonin and melatonin responsible for healthy sleep. Increasing the production of melatonin which is probably very useful as an oncostatic agent, especially in cases of breast or prostate cancer (Cos et al.1998; Neri et al. 1998).

Endorphins and enkephalins are secreted due to the yogic lifestyle which helps in detaching yourself from the various kinds of pains.

Effects of meditation show positive changes in ECG (electroencephalogram, heat waves), EMG (electromyogram, muscles waves) and increases skin resistance.

Creates a state of deep relaxation and reduces anxiety due to decreased levels of blood lactate (stress-related chemicals). It raises energy levels and strengthens the immune system.

Changes in gene expression through epigenetics, thus many types of cancer can be prevented. It can combat stress by changing the DNA (gene expression). A recent study confirms that apart from changes in hormone and brain functioning, stress can cause genetic changes. Evidence is there that chronic stress leads to disease by affecting gene expression. Dr. Perla Kaliman and her coworker scientists found that meditation can reverse the negative effects of stress.

Helps maintain telomere length. Longer telomeres help protect us from diseases.

Other Psychological benefits of Meditation-

- Helps retain the stability of the mind under adverse circumstances.
- Increases concentration and strengthens the mind.

- Increases tolerance power due to changes in one's belief system, attitude and behaviour.
- Improves memory. Thickens the grey matter of the brain.
- Increases the subjective feeling of happiness and contentment.

Positive metabolic effect of Meditation on Body-

- Improves proper coordination between all endocrine glands.
- Enhances the immune system. Research has revealed that meditation increases the activity of 'natural killer cells' that kill bacteria and cancer cells.
- Restores the normal rhythm of all endocrine glands, thus normalizing hormone levels.
- Improves cellular antioxidants which reduce the hazard of free radicals in the cell.
- Decreases muscle tension (any pain due to tension) and headaches.
- By keeping positive thoughts about your body you can change the physiology of the body for a healthier one.
- The visualization of the healing process over time has been proven to speed up the actual healing of the body.

I recollect reading about experiences shared by Vianna Stibal, an artist, writer and expert in Theta Healing. This naturopathy and diet practitioner developed bone cancer in the right leg and was advised amputation. She tried naturopathy, cleansing, diet, visualization and affirmations but did not see much recovery. She did theta meditation and commanded her body to heal immediately. Her leg which was shrunken 3 inches returned to normal size and she got cured.

The Pillars of Cellular Healing Meditation for Cancer-

Relaxation: Breaks tension and fear; help you accept your body as a **partner** in the healing process.

Self-awareness: Enables you to dig deep into your motivations, aspirations and distortions.

Positive mental status: Actively and positively influences the immune system.

Positive affirmations: Unlocks latent spiritual forces within and enhances healing.

Spiritual energy: The seven qualities of the soul are essential for the healing of every cell of the body. These can be increased by practising meditation.

Meditation for the caregiver and distant healing-

Meditation not only benefits "patients" but also deems useful for caregivers, medical and paramedical professionals, especially to manage and reduce their stress. Meditation changes your environment. Healing vibration to the patients can also be given by another individual like the caregiver or medical staff. I, along with other meditators, regularly do collective meditation for the healing of diseased patients. To top that, it also generates vibrations for self-healing. Meditation as medication at medical establishments improves the functioning and rates of recovery, as well as, reduces the cost of treatment with the comprehensive and holistic recovery of the client at all levels.

There are different types of meditation-

- Transcendental Meditation
- Zen Meditation
- Vipashyana
- Preksha
- Kundalini Jagran
- Saral Meditation
- Rajyoga by Patanjali
- Sudershan Kriya
- Mantra meditation
- Pranayam

- Rajyoga Meditation taught by Brahma Kumaris

I have been practising '**Rajyoga meditation**' (11) since 1986. I am writing in detail about this meditation specifically because it has helped me not only in healing but also in other aspects of life.

By practising Rajyoga, you become the ruler of your mind. It is the science and art of harmonizing spiritual, mental and physical energies by establishing a connection with the ultimate source of spiritual energy, the Supreme Soul, for enjoying an ever healthy, ever wealthy and ever happy life.

Definition of Rajyoga:

- Communion of the inner self with the Supreme.
- Tuning of the mind with the Supreme.
- Practice of higher consciousness.
- Self-development mental exercise.

How to use Rajyoga meditation in spiritual Healing?

As described previously in Chapter 7, healing starts from within and drawing upon the higher power is necessary for holistic healing.

Rajyoga meditation also has two components-

- Soul consciousness

- Supreme consciousness (connect with Supreme)

It is more accurate to say that Rajyog meditation is not just a meditation technique, but it is the art of living life. A meditative lifestyle can be described in three steps-

First step- How to practice Rajyoga meditation while sitting down? (morning and evening)

Second step- How to keep positive thoughts while performing actions? (Karma Yoga)

Third step- How to get the energy from things you consume during the day?

During Rajyoga meditation the practitioner remains awake and vigilant but the body enters a state of deep muscle relaxation.

The first step

For spiritual healing, sit down and charge your mind with Rajyoga meditation every morning and evening.

In the morning, our mind is fresh and the absorption capability of the subconscious mind is greater than what it is during the day. The moment you wake up, wish a very good morning to God, the Supreme Father, the Supreme Soul and create thoughts of self-respect by thinking - 'I am the Master Almighty, I am the child of the Supreme Being'.

Then immediately get out of your bed and head to a dedicated place for daily meditation.

The four stages of Rajyoga meditation are depicted in **Fig8.2**.

STAGES IN RAJYOGA

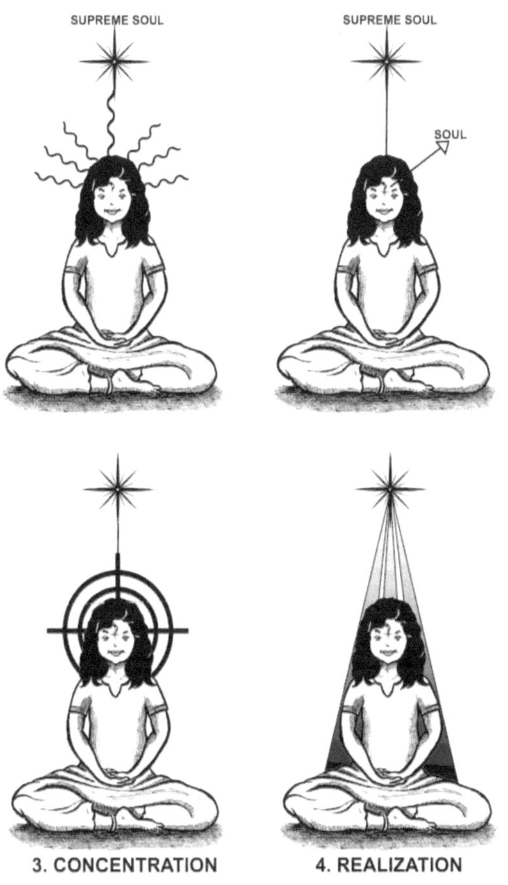

(Fig8.2)

Initiation- To begin, you make the decision to meditate and go to a dedicated meditation place or room. Sit comfortably and keep your back straight. It is not a chanting or a repeated prayer but an internal conversation and communion with the Supreme Soul. You are now ready for meditation.

Meditation- Withdraw your mind from the surroundings and turn it within, think and visualise yourself to be a soul. To get charged, establish yourself in a soul-conscious stage with the direction of the following statements -

'I am a soul... golden star-like energy... situated at the centre of my forehead, separate from this body that is my vehicle...
I am a being of peace... Loveful being... a being of light, a being of power...
I, the subtle being of light, can move beyond sound... beyond the physical world... beyond the sun, the moon and the stars...
In the beyond I become aware of another being, a living golden star-like energy of golden rays of light radiating from the Supreme star in all directions.
He is the ocean of peace... Ocean of love... Ocean of purity... the Almighty... Ocean of bliss...'

Concentration- Concentrate on the Supreme energy, the Almighty or the microconscient light.

'I am getting powerful energy from Him, just like SunLight... these are the healing energies...'

Realisation- In this stage, you are completely absorbed.

'I am getting healed... I am getting pure... I bathed... Now, I am now cleansed and purified... I feel free and light... and healed... refreshed by the Ocean.

Second step

Karma yoga- While performing karma (actions), remind yourself of powerful positive thoughts.

'I am healthy... I am a star of success... I can overcome obstacles... I am a being of peace and stability... I am an overflowing source of good wishes...I am spreading light and might to the world... my smile will work as a gift of greeting to everyone... I am working under the canopy of God'

Third step

Charge anything you consume, food, water or even medicines. Take whatever you are about to have in your hand and give it vibrations of positive thoughts and the rays of the Almighty God Father to purify it. Repeat these thoughts three to five times and make it a habit to charge every time before consuming anything. Food charged with these thoughts has tremendous power to heal your sickness and make you healthy **(Fig 8.3.)**

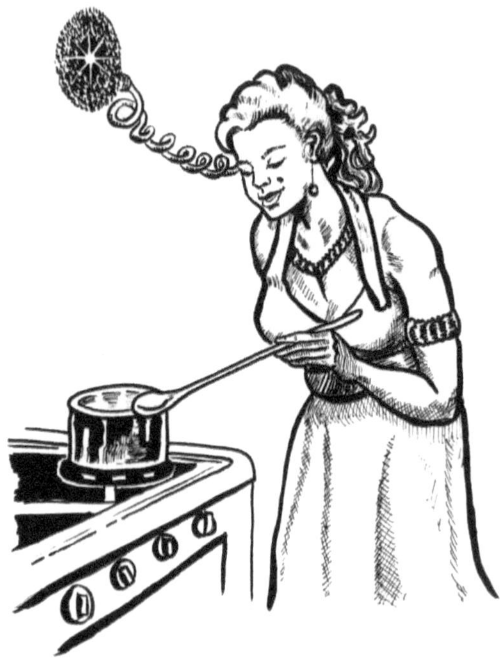

(Fig 8.3)

I practice Rajyoga meditation every day to keep hale and hearty. Readers are requested to carry out this healing with 100% faith and patience to see a positive result.

Summary

- Meditation is an ancient technique of self-healing. It should definitely be taught along with medicine.

- Meditation relieves acute and chronic stress which helps in healing the mind and body during illness.
- Meditation acts at a cellular level and reverses the process of the disease.
- Distant healing can be given to the patients by caregivers and medical professionals.

Chapter 9

Guided Rajyoga Healing Commentaries and Affirmations

"Meditation is the silent time to observe and remove the shadows of ego that blocks the light of love"

-Brahma Kumaris

In the previous chapter you learned that meditation is a journey of the self through the self, to the self. Meditation brings happiness in life and healing can be achieved by practising it regularly and sincerely. It is not just about mending your physical health, healing is required in various aspects of life. I have been practising and experiencing Rajayoga meditation since 1986. In this period filled with life's twists and turns, I have experimented with and leveraged it for various purposes. In this chapter, I have consolidated a variety of short meditation exercises for physical and emotional healing which can be practised easily.

Following the first step is necessary to practise meditation for any purpose.

Sit comfortably, keep your back straight... you can keep your eyes open or closed... do what makes you feel comfortable... withdraw your mind from the surroundings and focus your attention on your breath...

Take a few deep breaths, with every inhale visualise that positive energy of the universe is entering your body... and with each exhale you are relieving stress... low feeling... and negative energy... Focus your attention on the centre of the forehead...

Now read ahead, visualize and try to feel it. It will take some time to be able to practice this without the book. We have consolidated the audio/video meditation series on the YouTube channel –

Dr. Pushpa Pandey -
https://tinyurl.com/2p8w6u9n.

SOUL

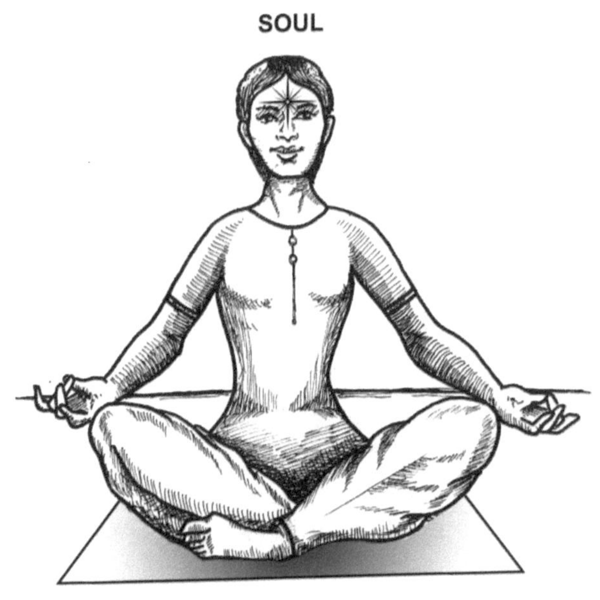

(Fig. 9.1)

For healing any diseased organ of the body-

I am a divine being... I am light... I have healing powers within... I reside in the centre of my forehead like a sparkling star, metaphysical energy. White powerful healing rays are emanating from the centre of my forehead, and spreading to my entire body... The brain, the face and the upper limbs are now getting filled with those white healing rays... Now, the healing rays are permeating through the heart... the lung... and the stomach... to the back... and to both the lower limbs... Every cell of the body is getting charged.

Now, visualise another point of light in front and above... He is the Supreme... He is just like the sun. Powerful healing rays... are emerging from Him and entering into my body, just like a laser beam... from the centre of my forehead to each and every cell. Now focus these beams on the diseased part and visualize (for 3-4 min)... Any blockages in this area are getting cleansed and replaced by healthy light... diseased cells are getting replaced by healthy cells... Now, I am light... I am healed... and I am healthy.

For relieving stress and anxiety

My body is relaxed... and comfortable... I am a peaceful being. Peace is my innate nature... Peaceful vibrations are emanating from the centre of my forehead, spreading to both the hemispheres of my brain... My brain has become peaceful... very peaceful... Now, peaceful vibrations are spreading to my face... I feel relaxed... My eyes are calm and at peace... These peaceful vibrations are spreading below the shoulder joints to both the hands... I am relaxed... My fingers have become light and peaceful... My heart is filled with a peaceful vibration... My heart rate has become normal... My respiratory rate has reduced... My heart is filled with peace... My back muscles are relaxed... The stomach is working normally... I am relaxed... Peaceful vibrations are spreading to my lower limbs... My calf muscles are relaxed... the lower limb is now relaxed and peaceful up to the toe... I am radiating peaceful vibrations in all directions.

I now visualise a point of light in front of me... that is the Ocean of Peace... Peaceful vibrations are falling upon me... I am absorbing them and diving deep into the ocean of peace... I am peaceful... relaxed... and filled with enthusiasm.

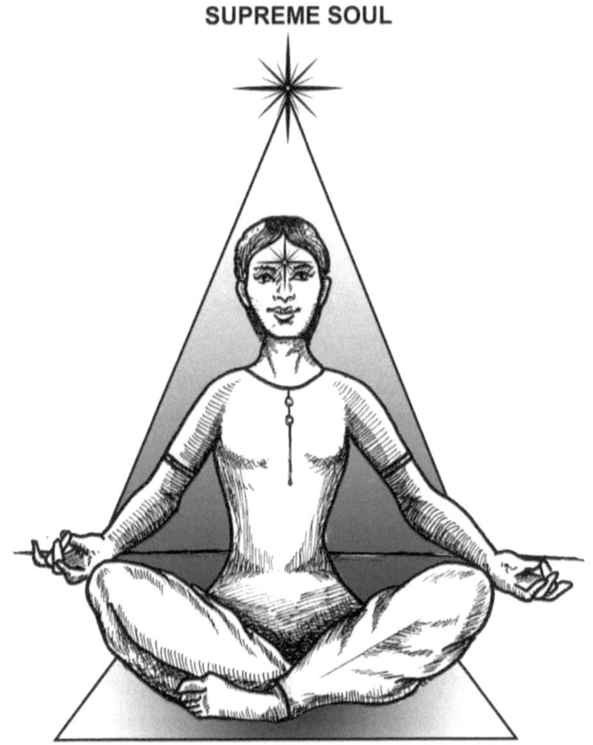

(Fig. 9.2)

For right karma

I am a wise being... I create my own destiny... I visualise myself as a shining star in the centre of my forehead... Powerful positive thoughts are emerging from the centre of my forehead and are spreading to my body... These positive thoughts are creating a positive environment... I accept every situation... Any person's bad behaviour towards me is a consequence of my past Karma... I am focusing on the present... I am creating the right energy, the right Karma... I am creating my present... I can visualise my Father, God, as a point of light... I am absorbing powerful energy from Him... I am performing every Karma in remembrance of... the Supreme Father... My destiny is secure... Now, I am a happy being... I am a healthy being.

For Improving Emotional Health

I am a loveful being... love... which is my innate quality... I am visualising myself as a loveful tiny point of light ... pure Love is emerging from the centre of the forehead ...and entering into each cell of my body... body cells are now in harmony... I love myself... I love my body... I love others ... The environment around me has become filled with pure Love... whoever comes into this environment is also feeling pure love... my negativity, hatred.. jealousy... anger have melted away in my own pure love... now I visualise my Supreme Father who is the ocean of love... I am receiving unconditional love from him as a shower... I am absorbed in the pure unconditional love of God... feel emotionally healthy...I have good feelings for everyone ... I treat everyone with royalty and dignity ...respect and loving detachment... my words are like a jewel of wisdom gently touching the soul who hears them ... My body is also getting healthy

Sleep Meditation- Free yourself from tension before going to bed.

Sit comfortably, take a few deep breaths and reflect on your day... Have I done anyone harm? If yes, visualise and ask for their forgiveness... If someone else has done you harm, forgive them... and surrender your worries to God...

Now go to your bed, lie down and relax your body from your toes to your head.

My feet are relaxed... calf muscles are relaxed... The sensation is moving upwards... Both the lower limbs have become so light that it feels as if they are absent... Back muscles are relaxed... Both the hands are by the side of the body... they have become light and relaxed... The sensation is moving upwards... My lungs and heart... are now relaxed... Below the neck... it feels as if there is no sensation... Face muscles are relaxed... Eyes are getting a heavy feeling... and becoming drowsy... All the sensation is limited to the centre of the forehead, like a small... shining star... I am a peaceful being... My brain has become peaceful and cool... Now I visualise the Supreme Father, the Ocean of peace, like another tiny star above my head... I feel peaceful vibrations coming towards me and encircling my bed... I am safe, fearless...

protected... and relaxed... I am feeling... drowsy... and now I am going to sleep.

For converting fear and negative feelings to positive feelings-

I am a powerful being... I am the creator of my own thoughts and destiny... I have complete control over my mind... Whatever happened in the past is history that taught me a lesson... Past is past, I am the creator of my new destiny... I am visualising myself as a powerful star... in the centre of my forehead... Powerful and purposeful thoughts are emanating from the centre of my head and spread to the entire body... I have become fearless... I can focus my thoughts on whatever and whenever I want to concentrate... And my body is now filled with positive vibrations... I am visualising the Almighty in front of me, who is a micro-conscient point of light like the sun... His powerful rays are coming towards me... I have become master almighty... and a pure... happy... fearless and.. blessed soul... I am safe... I am healed.

Distant healing meditation- This can be practised by the caretaker and other people who come in contact with the patient.

Sit back relaxed... After taking a few breaths... visualise a tiny star in the centre of your forehead...

From the star, powerful rays are emerging and filling my body... My body has become like an angel...

I visualise my Supreme Father, God, another point of light... I am getting healing vibrations from Him... I am filled with healing energy... Now, I am visualising the patient in front of me... and I am giving healing energy to them... they are getting better and better, their subtle body and gross body are now healed... They are happy and healthy...

This meditation can be done by a group or for a group of patients.

Just like your electronic gadgets, it's all about charging your batteries from the ultimate power source (the Supreme Soul). The charging takes time, meditation should be a constant process (Fig-9.3)

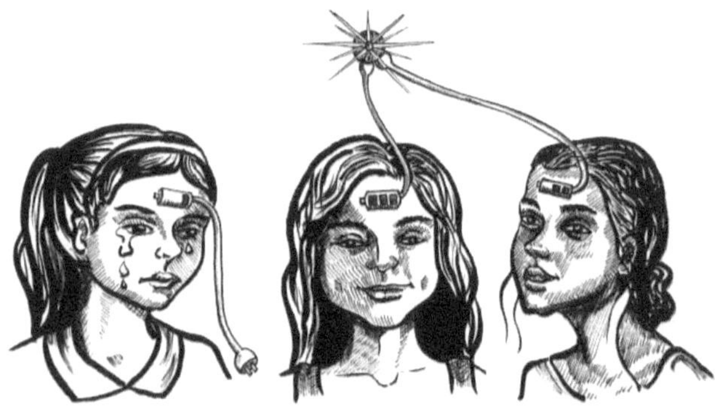

(Fig. 9.3)

Few affirmations which can be repeated 2-3 times every day to create positive energy and promote healing-

- I am a peaceful being, I radiate peace to my entire body
- I am a loveful being, I radiate love to everyone
- I am a blissful being, I am a blessed soul
- I am a powerful being, I radiate positivity to everyone
- I am a pure being, I radiate purity to my body and to everyone
- I am always happy
- I am healthy, all my family members are healthy
- My body is healthy
- My immune system is good, I am healed
- Everyone is good
- I radiate love to every cell of my body
- I am victorious, I am successful, success is my birthright
- I am a lucky being
- My mind is my best friend
- God is with me always
- I am honest and simple
- All my relatives are very cooperative
- I am very easy
- I am God's child, my future is secure
- I am fearless
- I am enough
- I am light
- I am serene
- I am contented
- I am stable and unhurt

- I am an angel
- God has chosen me to bestow happiness and health
- My anger has converted into assertion
- My nature of blaming others has turned into responsibility
- My nature of comparing myself with others has changed into being contented
- I respect myself, I respect everyone
- I value time, I complete my task before time, I respect everyone's time

Affirmations while drinking water or cooking and eating food

- The water I am drinking has pure energy
- Water is like nectar healing my body
- Water is detoxifying my body
- I appreciate my kitchen which is an a nourishment centre
- I am grateful to all the food that supports my health
- I love spending time in kitchen
- Food is *Prasad* and full of godly power
- I choose healthy food
- My family loves to eat healthy food
- The food I consume keeps my body healthy

Section 3
Preventing the Preventable

"Prevention is a very important part of solving the problem of cancer"

-Eva Vertis

As I started writing this section, I received a call from a local engineering college to deliver a session on "Awareness of Cancer in Women". Initially, the intended target audience of this book was women over 30, however, after this call, I realized the importance of the preventive aspect of cancer, especially for younger females.

In the previous chapters, we learned the importance of a healthy diet, exercise and stress management during pregnancy. If expectant mothers take care of these three points, the chances of cancer are greatly reduced in their babies. Most of the non-communicable diseases like diabetes and cancer are thought to be of fetal origin. Although the disease occurs in adulthood, the cause may be environmental factors in the womb. This is called the "fetal origin of adult disease". Only 5-10% are found to be genetic cancer, the more common are lifestyle diseases.

There are two chapters in this section. The first chapter covers some of the preventive strategies and a few screening methods for cervical health of the uterus which is usually ignored by women. The second chapter, authored by onco-surgeon Dr. Preeti Jain, talks about breast awareness. It is in a questionnaire format covering the most common questions that have been asked in our programs.

"Woman empowerment is the first step in making this world heaven."

Chapter 10

Is your Uterus Healthy?

"We have forgotten that curing cancer starts with preventing cancer in the first place."

-David Agus

Uterus is a reproductive organ of the female genital system. An unhealthy uterus can cause many problems in a woman's lifetime, however, in this chapter, we will only discuss ways to prevent cancer of the uterus.

Following are the most commonly asked questions-

Q1- What is cancer?

Ans- Cancer is a group of diseases characterized by uncontrolled cell division leading to the growth of abnormal tissue and spread to other organs.

Q2- Doctor, tell me about the signs and symptoms that I should be aware of to prevent cancer of the uterus?

Ans-

- No symptoms in early stage
- Abnormal white discharge
- Inter menstrual bleeding - Spotting or bleeding in between normal menses
- Contact bleeding
- Postmenopausal bleeding
- Back pain and leg pain
- Loss of weight and appetite

Q3- Doctor, you mentioned earlier that there are no symptoms in the initial stages of cancer. Can you tell me the methods to identify if my uterus is healthy?

Ans- In order to identify a healthy uterus, you need to first understand that there are two types of cancers of the uterus -

- Carcinoma of cervix
- Carcinoma of the body of uterus

Carcinoma of cervix

Q4- What is a cervix? Which part of carcinoma is more common at what age?

Ans- Uterus has two parts- the mouth of the uterus is called the cervix and the upper part is known as the body of the uterus. Carcinoma cervix is more common from a young age upto any age, especially in developing countries like

India. Carcinoma body uterus is more common in developed countries like America and usually occurs after or around menopause.

Q5- Can cancer cervix be cured completely?

Ans- Yes, if diagnosed early-

- Symptoms start at a younger age and it takes 10 years to become cancer.
- If treated early, it can be cured completely but if not treated, it can progress to cancer.
- Regular check-up is necessary to detect premalignant lesions.

Q6- What are the risk factors for carcinoma of the cervix?

Ans-

- Sexually active at an early age.
- Multiple sexual partners.
- Childbirth at an early age.
- Multiple pregnancies.
- Smoking.
- Having a partner who has multiple sexual partners.

Q7- Who gets carcinoma cervix?

Ans- 99% of cases of cervical cancer (or carcinoma cervix) are due to HPV (human papillomavirus 16 and 18)

- It is a viral infection.
- HPV is the main cause.
- Virus is transmitted by sexual activity.
- Women who are sexually active can get the virus infection and cancer.
- A few women are more prone than others.

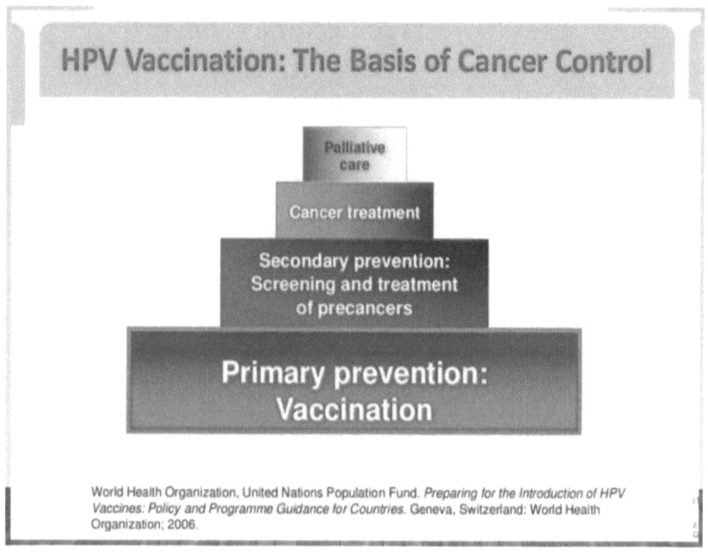

(Fig 10.1)

Q8- Is there any vaccine to prevent cervical cancer?

Ans- Two vaccines are available against HPV which is the most common cause of cervical cancer.

HPV vaccines are highly effective in preventing the infection of susceptible women with the HPV types covered by the vaccine. HPV vaccine should be given to females before they reach an age when the risk of HPV infection increases and they are at subsequent risk of cervical cancer. The HPV vaccine can be given to all females between 9 to 45 years.

For 15-year-olds and younger, only two doses are recommended, the second dose should be 6-12 months apart. Over 15 years, 3 doses are recommended.

Cervarix- 0-1-6 months (over 15 years of age), i.e. second dose after one month and third dose after six months.

Gardasil- 0-2-6 months (over 15 years of age), i.e. second dose after two months and third dose after six months.

Q9- What is the meaning of a screening test? What are the methods for regular screening of cervical health?

Ans- A healthy person having no symptoms undergoes a screening test to detect precancerous problems. The tests include-

- HPV testing every 5 years after 30 years of age in India.

USPSTF RECOMMENDATION FOR ROUTINE CERVICAL CANCER SCREENING	
Population	Recommendation
Aged less than 21 year (pap-smpar)	No Screening
Aged less than 21 to 29 year	Anyone of the following • Cytology alone every 3 years • HPV Testing alone every 5 years • Co testing HPV Cytology every 5 years
Aged greater than 65 year	No Screening after adequate negative prior screening results
Hysterectomy with removal of cervix	No screening in individual who do not have history of high grade cervical precancerous reason or cervical cancer
US PREVENTIVE SERVICES TASK FORCE (*USPSTF)*	

(Table 10.1)

- 2. Pap smear (cytology test) every 3 years. In India screening starts at 30 years.
- 3. VIA testing

Q10- What is the Pap test (cytology)? How is it done?

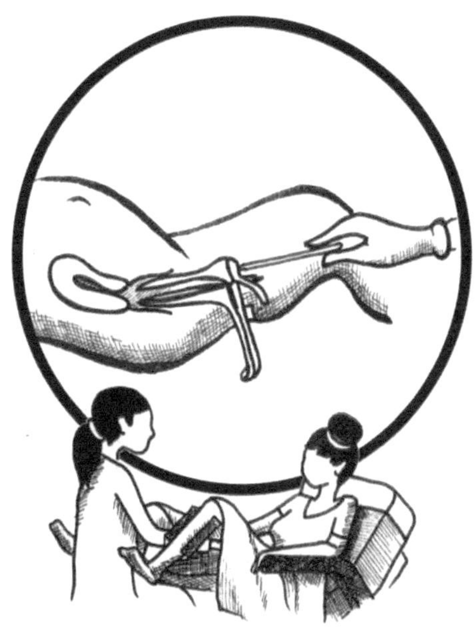

(Fig. 10.2)

Ans- Pap smear, also called a Pap test, is a screening test for detecting pre-cancer or cervical cancer in women.

In a Pap test, the doctor uses a vaginal speculum to hold vaginal walls apart to see the cervix. Next, a sample of cells from the cervix is collected using a small cone-shaped brush and a tiny plastic spatula.

There are two methods of cytology-

- Conventional
- Liquid-based cytology (LBC recent and more accurate)

Q11- What is HPV testing? How is it done?

Ans- **99% of cervical cancers are due to the HPV virus**. The HPV test is a screening test for cervical cancer. This test does not identify if there is cancer, instead, it detects the presence of HPV, the virus that causes cervical cancer. Certain types of HPV — including types 16 and 18 — increase your cervical cancer risk. HPV home test kits are also readily available for females from 30 years of age.

Q12- What is the VIA test?

Ans- Visual inspection with acetic acid (VIA)

This is a simple and inexpensive test for the detection of cervical precancerous lesions and early invasive cancer. The results of the VIA test are immediately available and do not require any laboratory support.

Q13- What is colposcopy and when is it done?

Ans- Colposcopy is not a screening method. Doctors recommend this test when abnormal findings are detected in any screening test. It is used to find cancerous or abnormal cells that can become cancerous in the cervix, vagina, or vulva. These abnormal cells are sometimes called "precancerous tissue". A colposcopy also looks for other health conditions, such as genital warts or noncancerous growths called polyps.

Carcinoma of Body of Uterus-

Q14- What are the signs and symptoms of carcinoma body uterus?

Ans-

- Post-menopausal bleeding
- 45 years or older, or menopausal having heavy, prolonged bleeding (more than 8 days) or frequent menses (less than 21 days)
- Younger than 45 years, obese, with abnormal bleeding even after a medical treatment
- Pap smear, shows endometrial cells after menopause
- White discharge

Q15- What is menopause?

Ans- Menopause is the natural stopping of a woman's menstrual cycle. It marks the permanent cessation of reproductive fertility. Spontaneous menopause is recognised to have occurred after 12 months of amenorrhoea (usually from 45-55 years).

Q16- What is perimenopause?

Ans- It is the period immediately before and upto 1 year after the final menstrual period. It may last for 3-5 years.

Q17- What is postmenopause?

Ans- It is the span of time dating from the final menstrual period.

Q18- What is postmenopausal bleeding?

Ans- It is bleeding that occurs 12 months after the last normal period. However, it is recommended that any vaginal bleeding that occurs after 6 months after the last period (presumed menopause) should be investigated

Q19- Is every postmenopausal bleeding cancer?

Ans- No, in 90% of the cases it is due to hormonal imbalance or some other benign cause.

Q20- Is there a screening method to detect carcinoma uterus?

Ans- No, there are no routine investigations, but if anyone has symptoms then sonography and endometrial biopsy are taken.

Q21- How do I know that findings are normal or abnormal?

Ans- The doctor will inform you based on the sonography findings of the inner lining of the uterus, i.e. the endometrium. After menopause, a thin 3 to5 mm lining is considered normal.

A biopsy report also shows if the endometrial thickness is normal or abnormal (simple or atypical).

Q22- What are the risk factors for carcinoma of the uterus?

Ans-

- Obesity
- Increased waist to hip ratio
- Taller than average height
- Type 1 and type 2 diabetes
- Hypertension
- Polycystic ovarian syndrome
- Early menarche (age of first menses)
- Late menopause
- Nulliparity (women who were never pregnant)
- Unopposed estrogen therapy
- Genetic
- Unhealthy lifestyle and physical inactivity
- Western diet
- Tamoxifen therapy

Q23- Doctor, I have heard about hysteroscopy. What is it?

Ans- Hysteroscopy is a procedure in which examination of the inside uterus is done by a thin light instrument in many medical problems. It is also the 'gold standard' for biopsy in carcinoma uterus investigations.

Q24- Doctor can you briefly tell me about a healthy lifestyle, especially during menopause?

Have a healthy diet- more coloured fruits, vegetables, no fast or fried food and proper hydration is necessary. Calcium-rich diet, milk, curd or yoghurt, methi, ragi etc. Extra calcium 1000-1500mg should be taken to prevent osteoporosis.

Exercise enough- 150 minutes of aerobic exercise in a week, stretching and strength training 2-3 times a week.

Sleep well- deep sleep improves the immune system of the body

Adopt a stress-free life- through meditation, music, positive thinking

Summary

- Cancer cervix is preventable if screened regularly, and can be cured completely if diagnosed early
- 99% of the causes of cervical cancer are HPV 16-18 viruses. HPV vaccination

prevents HPV infection and cancer cervix.

- Postmenopausal bleeding should never be ignored and should be investigated properly.

Chapter 11

Awareness is Power: Breast Awareness

-Dr. Preeti Jain

Q1- What is the meaning of Breast awareness?

Ans- It is about becoming familiar with the breasts and the way they change throughout a woman's life. It is a concept that encourages women to know how their breasts look and feel normally so that they gain confidence about noticing any change which might help detect breast cancer early. Breast awareness as a concept is gaining increasing acceptance worldwide.

Changes in the breast that one should be aware of:

- Painless lump or thickening that feels different from the rest of the breast
- Change in size - it may be that one breast has become noticeably larger or noticeably lower.
- Recent retraction of the nipple.
- Rash on or around the nipple.
- Bloodstained spontaneous discharge from one or both the nipples.

- Puckering or dimpling of the skin overlying the breast.
- Swelling under the armpit or around the collarbone (where the lymph nodes are located).
- Constant pain in one part of the breast or armpit.

The 5-point code of Breast Awareness

- Know what is normal for you
- Know what changes to look and feel for
- Look and feel
- Report any changes to your doctor without delay
- Have a mammogram (x-ray of the breast) at least once in 2 years from the age of 40 (ideally every year)

*REF-Raghuram, Be breast aware, early detection saves lives, pink conns UBF ion, vol4 issue 4, May-July 18

Q2- What are the different diseases of the breast? What are their symptoms?

Ans- The common diseases involving the breast are infections, fibrocystic disease, benign and malignant tumours.

Breast infections

Generally occur in women who are breastfeeding. Sometimes bacterial infections lead to the accumulation of pus in the breast called an abscess. This is a very painful condition, often associated with fever. May need treatment with surgical drainage and antibiotics. Tuberculosis also affects breasts. Symptoms are similar to other breast infections however it needs treatment with antitubercular drugs.

Fibrocystic disease

Having pain or heaviness in the breasts before periods is common. However, in extreme cases, painful cysts form in the breast.

Benign lumps or fibroadenomas

They are commonly occurring lumps in the breasts of young females. They are largely harmless. They need surgical removal if they are large.

Breast cancer

Breast cancer is the most common cancer in women in India. It accounts for 27% of all cancers in women. Due to a lack of awareness and the absence of an organized population-based breast cancer screening, more than 70% of women present with the disease in advanced stages.

Symptoms of Breast cancer:

- Lump or thickening in the breast

- Nipple that is pulled in or changed in position or shape
- A rash on or around the nipple
- Bloodstained discharge
- Puckering or dimpling of skin
- Pain in the breast or armpit
- Change in size

Q 2.1- Who is at risk of Breast cancer?

Breast cancer doesn't have a single well-defined cause. However several risk factors have been identified that increase the risk of breast cancer. Some of the important risk factors are as follows.

Increasing age

- Nulliparity: The risk of breast cancer is higher in women who never produced any children.
- Family History
- Only 5 to 10% of breast cancers are familial.
- Menarche before 13 years: four-fold increase
- Menopause after 55 years: twice the incidence as compared to under 44 years
- Duration of menstruation > 30 years has higher risk
- First child before 19 years, half the risk compared to nulliparous

- Hormone Replacement Therapy (HRT) in postmenopausal women.
- Oral contraceptives for more than 10 years may increase the risk
- Obesity increases the risk of breast cancer

Q 2.2- How to reduce Breast cancer Risk

Ans-

- Prolonged breastfeeding
- Regular physical activity
- Weight control
- Avoidance of harmful use of alcohol
- Avoidance of exposure to tobacco smoke
- Avoidance of prolonged use of hormones
- Avoidance of excessive radiation exposure
- Perform breast self-examination regularly
- Physical breast exam by physician
- Follow recommended guidelines for mammograms
- Exercise regularly

Q3- My mother died of breast cancer. What are my chances of getting it? Is breast cancer genetic?

Ans- Only 5-10% of breast cancers are genetically transmitted and they present differently. Genetically transmitted cancers present at an early age, in the 30s or 40s, multiple blood relatives are affected, there may be many breast and ovarian cancers in the family or there may be breast and ovarian cancers in the same person also. These are due to genes called BRCA1 and BRCA2. If you have a strong family history, one can get tested for these genes however it should be done only after consultation with an oncologist. In case of BRCA positive status, one has to be under close surveillance with an oncologist who will advise more intense screening from time to time.

Q4-What are the methods of Breast screening?

Ans- Screening tests are performed on healthy individuals to look for signs of disease in women without symptoms. They should be part of every healthy woman's routine.

Screening modalities are as follows:

- Clinical breast examination - by a doctor once a year
- Breast self-examination - once a month
- Mammogram - once a year
- The following additional tests are performed based on the findings of screening tests:

- Breast USG
- MRI
- Thermography
- Tissue sampling
- BRCA testings

Q5- How is the Self-breast examination done?

Ans- Breast self-exam, or regularly examining your breasts on your own can be an important way to find breast cancer early when it is more likely to be treated successfully. The method involves the woman herself looking at and feeling each breast for possible lumps, distortions or swelling. It is a regular and repetitive monthly self-examination of the breast performed by a woman at the same time each month, preferably after the completion of menstruation each month.

Breast Self-Exam

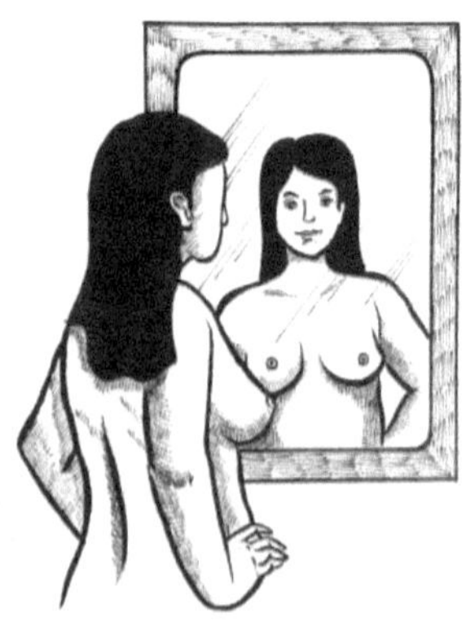

Step 1: Begin by looking at your breasts in the mirror with your shoulders straight and your arms on your hips. Here's what you should look for:

- *Notice the usual size, shape, and skin colour of your breasts.*

- *If you see any of the following changes, bring them to your doctor's attention:*
    - *Any visible distortion or swelling*
    - *Dimpling, puckering or bulging of the skin*
    - *A nipple that has changed position or an inverted nipple (pushed inward instead of sticking out)*
    - *Redness, soreness, rash, or swelling*

Step 2: *Now, raise your arms and look for the same changes.*

Step 3: *While you're at the mirror, look for any signs of fluid coming out of one or both nipples (this could be a watery, milky, or yellow fluid or blood).*

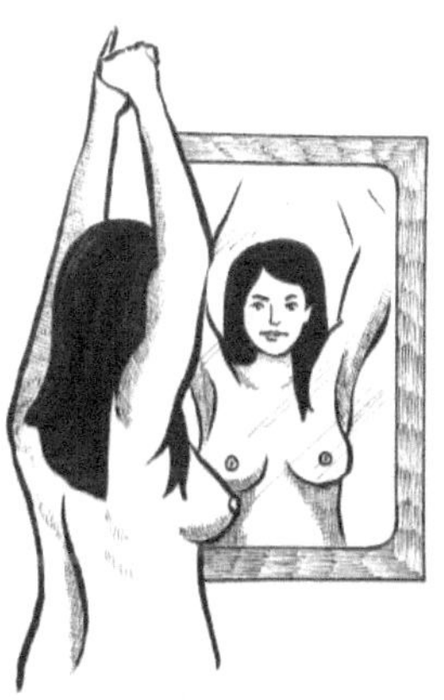

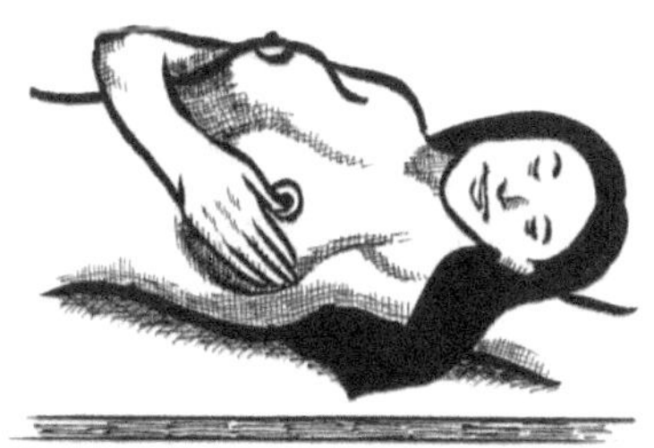

Step 4: *Next, feel your breasts while lying down, using your right hand to feel your left breast and then your left hand to feel your right breast. Use a*

firm, smooth touch with the first few finger pads of your hand, keeping the fingers flat and together. Use a circular motion, about the size of a quarter.

Cover the entire breast from top to bottom, side to side - from your collarbone to the top of your abdomen, and from your armpit to your cleavage.

Follow a pattern to be sure that you cover the whole breast. You can begin at the nipple, moving in 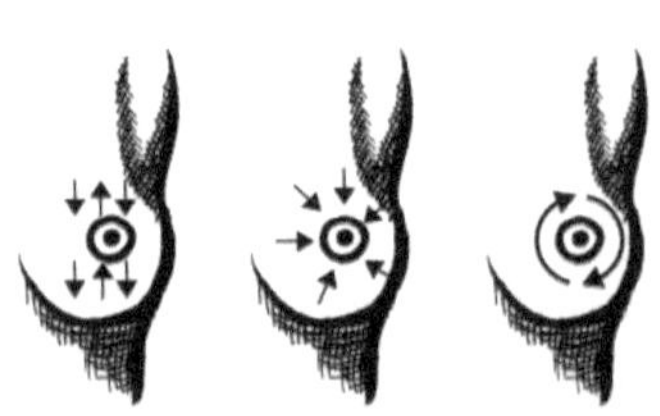 *larger and larger circles until you reach the outer edge of the breast. You can vary the pressure applied by your fingers and feel the most superficial or the deeper tissues.*

Step 5: *Finally, feel your breasts while you are standing or sitting. Many women find that the easiest way to feel their breasts is when their skin is wet and slippery, so they like to do this step in the shower. Cover your entire breast, using the same hand movements described in the previous step.*

Clinical Breast exam is an examination of the breast by a doctor or other health professional. The doctor will carefully feel the breasts and under the arms for lumps or anything else that seems unusual. It should be done every 1-3 years starting at the age of 20 years and every year starting at the age of 40. It is recommended more frequently if one has a strong family history of breast cancer. Breast examinations are best performed soon after the menstrual period.

Q6- What is a screening mammogram? If I can not feel a lump why should I have a mammogram?

Ans- A screening mammogram (x-ray of the breast) is done to detect breast lumps in an impalpable stage when neither the lady nor the doctor can feel a lump in the breast.

A mammogram is an effective breast screening method to detect breast cancer many years before it actually shows up. Early detection of breast cancer offers the best chance for a successful treatment. It is advisable and necessary to do a screening mammogram once every two years from the age of 40.

Q7- Is it safe to have a mammogram? Does it cause a radiation hazard?

Ans- It is indeed safe mammography involves a tiny dose of radiation; the risk to health from this is insignificant. The radiation dose delivered during a mammography is similar to the one you receive during a dental X-Ray.

Q8- Is mammography painful?

While mammography may cause momentary discomfort it should not be painful if it is done by a properly trained radiographer. With digital mammography, the discomfort is even less.

Myths and facts about cancer

Myth 1: Cancer is incurable.

Fact: Breast cancer can be cured if detected and treated in the early stages. The cure rate is as high as 95% in the early stage. That is why we emphasize awareness and screening so that more and more women can be diagnosed and treated at an early stage and achieve complete cures.

Myth 2: Cancer can be contagious. It spreads from one person to another.

Fact: Cancer doesn't spread to others by any type of contact.

Myth 3: Breast cancer runs in the family.

Fact: Only 5-10 % of breast cancers are familial. Rest all are sporadic.

Myth 4: Cancer causes pain from the beginning.

Fact: Cancer is painless, to begin with. It gets painful only in the advanced stages.

Myth 5: Wearing a black bra or a tight bra can cause breast cancer.

Fact: Wearing any type of undergarment doesn't affect your chances of cancer.

Myth 6: A Biopsy of a needle test can lead to the spreading of cancer.

Fact: Any type of procedure including surgery can never lead to the spread or speeding up of cancer growth. The rate of growth and spread of cancer is the inherent property of cancer cells. It can not be changed by any biopsy test or surgery.

Myth 7: Cancer is a death sentence.

Fact: Most cancers of the body can be cured if diagnosed and treated in the early stages. Cancer can be treated even in advanced stages. However, the chances of cure and long term survival reduce as the disease stage advances.

Myth 8: Chemotherapy causes many side effects.

Fact: This was true when enough supportive medication was not available in the past. Nowadays we have very effective medicines that can control all side effects and make chemotherapy a comfortable experience.

Myth 9: Chemotherapy leads to permanent hair loss.

Fact: The hair loss caused by chemotherapy is only temporary. All hair comes back once treatment is stopped.

Myth 10: Breast removal is a part of breast cancer treatment.

Fact: Removal of breasts is not necessary in all cases. In most cases nowadays, breasts can be preserved. Reconstruction of the breast is possible even after complete removal.

Chapter 12

Golden principles of Stress free-Life

"No body is defeated until he starts blaming somebody else"

-John wooden, Basketball coach

You have learned in previous chapters about different dimensions of life and ways to make your life healthy. This chapter is like the last ritual of this healing *yajna* that you can take as a *prasad* (gift) in the form of 15 principles for a stress-free life.

Psychosomatic problems are spiralling in the 21st century. Stress and anxiety are the mothers of all illnesses and it has been estimated that 55% of health problems are psychosomatic in nature. To lead a stress-free life you can revise these principles of life in your daily routine

Stress = Pressure of the circumstances / Capacity or strength to face

The pressure of the circumstances cannot be reduced because the external situations and people are not in your control. However, you can increase your inner strength and capacity to face the situation.

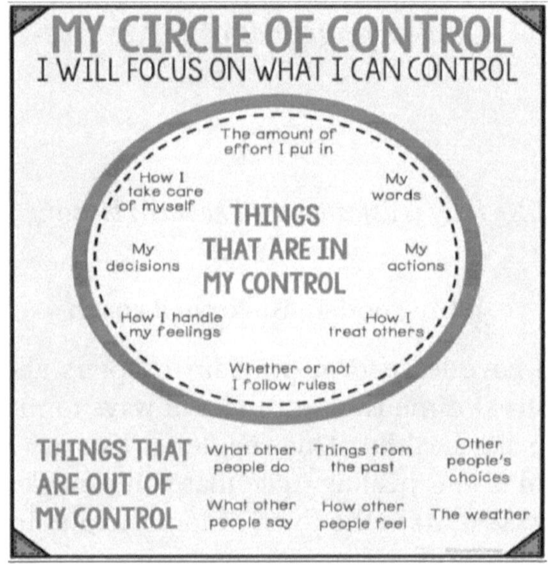

1. The first step to getting out of stress and anxiety is to become aware of your stress and anxiety. **Stress** is a form of pain that comes to tell us that there is something we need to **change**. **Pain** is a messenger that comes to tell us that there is something we need to **learn**.

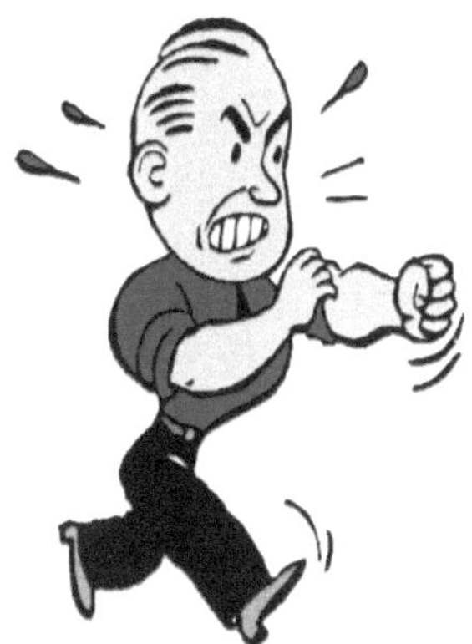

2. Every situation in our lives presents some direct or indirect advantages. Make it a habit to ponder over those advantages, however small they may be.

3. Keep your self-esteem high. No matter what anyone says or does, you can respond positively, you do not need to get upset because you value yourself. You believe in yourself - I am a powerful being, I am a blissful being, I am a special soul, I am a fortunate soul.

4. Perform every action in a soul-conscious stage. Remember God while performing every karma.

5. Have an attitude of gratitude. Make a list of attainments in life and be happy

6. Renounce your desires, JHAL - jealousy, hatred, anger, lust and leg-pulling.

7. Don't feel inferior by comparing yourself with others. Remember that

there is no one else like you in this entire world.

8. Forgive and forget- Forget all those people who have created hurdles in your life and made it more difficult to live. Until you take this positive step you won't be able to forget all those unhappy and painful incidents.

9. Whenever possible, spare some time to help others by rendering your services to others. This giving attitude will definitely minimize your worries, tensions and anxiety.

10. Perform karma for the benefit of others. Pray for the success of others and enjoy others' successes.

11. This world is a huge drama and we are all actors playing the specific roles allotted to each of us. Accept everyone as they are and don't feel anxious by observing any co-actor's roles. Remain comfortable when others do not act according to your desire, <u>still better response is to enjoy</u> the different behaviours of fellow actors.

12. Past is history, the future is a mystery and the present is a gift for you. Focus on the present.

13. Lead a balanced life. Take sattvic vegetarian food, walk regularly, wake up before sunrise and get sufficient sleep –

discipline in life will keep your mind and body healthy and stress-free.

14. Become trusty, surrender every relation and everything to God. Surrender the result of every action to God

15. Learn Meditation and master your mind. If you want to join the meditation group, mail me at drpushpapandey@gmail.com.

Be Healthy - Be happy - Be holy - Be yogi
Make your life and the lives of others like diamonds'

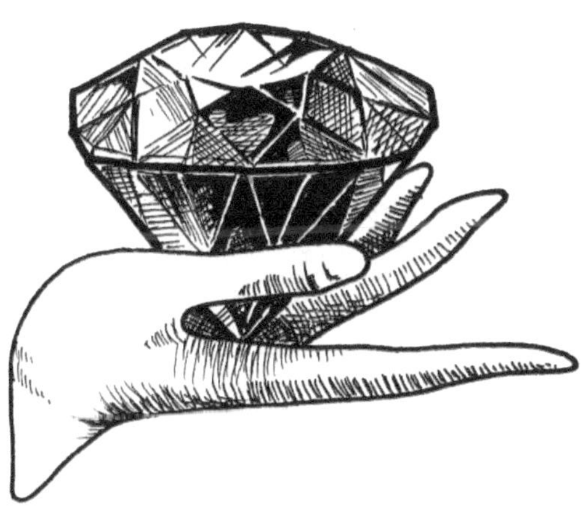

'

About the Author

Dr. Pushpa Pandey MD is a senior gynecologist at the Bombay hospital, Jabalpur, Madhya Pradesh, India. She has an experience of 40 years of gynecological practice. She has contributed a lot to the welfare of women in society and has received the 'Women Empowerment Award' in the year 2015 by the Federation of Obstetrics and Gynecological Society of India. She has a keen interest in spiritualism and has been practicing Rajyoga meditation since 1986. Every day she teaches meditation to the general public, her patients, and even other medical professionals. She is a good orator and conducts many programs on stress-free living, cancer, Rajyoga meditation and Bhagavad Gita in many universities, colleges, and for the public in and around India. She is a good combination of science and spirituality. She believes that for achieving good health, medication should be combined with meditation. She has done an immense amount of research on the knowledge of the Bhagavad Gita. She has also authored many books on stress-free life, Bhagavad Gita, high-risk pregnancy and Garbh sanskar, and has worked tirelessly to transform thousands of lives for the better.

Testimonials

really listen to my body and mind, feel all the feelings so I can lead a healthy lifestyle and proactively take care of my body and health.

- Shalini, Global director of instruction, generation: you employed

Excellent combination of science and spirituality. 'Medicine to Meditation' will bring about great faith in cancer patients and build their strength to fight out the malady with good vibes and vigor. This is an exemplary biography of the author's stint with endometrial cancer. It will help find positivity in all negative situations.

- Dr. Bhagyalaxmi Nayak, MD, FICOG, PhD, PG
Dept. of Gynae Oncology, Regional Cancer Center, Cuttack,
Vice-president, AOGIN, India
Chairperson CME Committee AGOI
Asst. Editor Indian Journal of Gynae Oncology
Peer Reviewer Indian Journal of Surgical Oncology

This book illuminates the ideal melange of spiritualism and healing through positive stoking. Coming from a practitioner of Rajyoga who beat back a cancer bout through optimistic approach is a must read for generations across the spectrum for healthy living, especially so in the fast paced world today. I am really grateful to the author for sharing her rich experience for the benefit of humankind in the long run. A must read for all who wish to be more conscious in their way of living.

- Lt Gen Upendra Dwivedi, AVSM, General Officer Commanding in Chief (GOC - in - C), Northern Command, Indian Army

These are testing times, times of uncertainty and turmoil. A time when most of us are engulfed by the fearful thoughts of sufferings and illnesses, either for ourselves or for our loved ones. The present COVID era has definitely increased these feelings of fear and despair, even manifold. So, in these testing times, this book comes as a breath of fresh air and forces us to rethink our way of living and level of positivity. This is truly a story of the journey...

From fear to Faith...
From medicine to meditation...
From despair to positivity...
A must read for all of us.

- Dr Shruti S Agrawal
Mrs India MIQS 2017 Title winner.
Pageant grooming coach &
Corporate trainer in Health & Wellness.

This book presents great insights for living a healthy life. Rare to find the medical and spiritual intersection.

Surbhi Gupta, Product Manager, Facebook, California USA

'Medicine to meditation' is an eye opener for the physicians, nurses and health professionals who are reclaiming the title of the 'Healer'. The author has explored the missing dimension of medicine on how the power of mind helps in **healing** *of the body and beyond. There is no doubt that during the healing process, practice of Rajyoga meditation works like an antioxidant. It not only increases the will power of the patients to fight the disease but also reduces its gravity. This book is a novel approach to enlighten the mind of innumerable cravers of knowledge and help them to take the 'QUANTUM leap' in their career and lives, along with positive changes in intellect and thoughts. With my personal experience in this Rajyoga meditation, I can ascertain that it is easier to deal with frustrating and irritating situations in life.*

- Prof Dr. Madhu Jain, Ex-HOD Dept. obs and gynae, BHU, Varanasi India

It is an awesome book, written in a very simple language which is easily understable by even the non-medicos. It truly clears all your doubts and fears which revolve around cancer diagnosis and treatment. It also provides you with a very clear vision not only of the disease, but also of health and spirituality. It is a must read for all, especially women of all ages as the story is very much relatable to every woman.

- Dr. Anamika, Associate Professor Ophthalmology, Rewa India

'Medicine to Meditation' is simple, inspirational, scientific and close to heart. The role of meditation in healing is described in an easily-understood way. This book is useful for everyone. As a gynecology cancer surgeon, I would like to emphasize that every woman should follow the screening methods and preventive measures to keep their uterus healthy. I wish everyone a healthy and peaceful life ahead.

- Dr. Kavita N Singh MS, PHD, Prof and Head of dept of obs and gynae, NSCB medical college Jabalpur, India

Amazing book! It is well-written and easy to understand. It broadens our understanding revolving around cancer diagnosis, its treatments, and the role of spirituality to overcome the challenges that come along with it. The topics discussed in the book are of huge relevance and should be known and talked about worldwide. I would love it if this book was more well known so more people can be exposed to this gem of a book.

-Sonal Sahu
Associate Director, Department of Finance and Accounting
Tecnológico de Monterrey, Campus Guadalajara
Mexico

The book is very interesting and informative, everyone should read it. The language is very simple, elaborate and easily graspable. We women at some point in our lives face similar emotional situations and conundrums as the author. The book teaches us how to handle such emotional aspects of life. It shares good knowledge of dealing with cancer and its treatment. Affirmations, visualizations, and meditation make us spiritually strong, so read the book and benefit yourself.

- Dr Anita Mishra, Gynecologist, Ghaziabad

Keep Connected

Youtube – *Dr. Pushpa Pandey*

Facebook- *pushpa.pandey.7146*

www.ingramcontent.com/pod-product-compliance
Lightning Source LLC
La Vergne TN
LVHW040726170726
843469LV00079B/984